P9-DBP-876

THE CHILD BEFORE BIRTH

LINDA FERRILL ANNIS

CORNELL UNIVERSITY PRESS | ITHACA AND LONDON

First published 1978 by Cornell University Press.
Published in the United Kingdom by Cornell University Press Ltd.,
2-4 Brook Street, London W1Y 1AA.
First printing, Cornell Paperbacks, 1978

International Standard Book Number (cloth) 0-8014-1039-8, (paper) 0-8014-9168-1
Library of Congress Catalog Card Number 77-3112
Printed in the United States of America by Vail-Ballou Press, Inc.
Librarians: Library of Congress cataloging information appears on the last page of the book.

TO DAVID AND MY PARENTS

Contents

Contents

Illustrations

Preface

This book provides a concise and general introduction to the many factors influencing the unborn child during the nine months from its conception to birth. There is helpful material here for those who work with young people as counselors, social workers, drug therapists, nutritionists, or medical advisers; for the young girl just reaching the age of sexual maturity who wonders about the birth process; for the young couple who think of themselves as potential parents and want to know what happens during each month of the development period; and for the newly pregnant woman who seeks insight into the process going on in her body. There is information, too, for any person (male or female) who may be concerned about the genetic transmission of defects or the effects of drugs and disease on the unborn child; the parents of a defective child may find an explanation for their situation, and in some instances reassurance for risking a second pregnancy, by learning of medical techniques that are used to circumvent possible damage.

The Child before Birth might be used in human growth and development courses and in child psychology courses offered in such departments as psychology, educational psychology, and sociology. Students in anatomy and physiology will also find the book useful.

LINDA FERRILL ANNIS

Plainsboro, New Jersey

THE CHILD BEFORE BIRTH

1 Introduction to
Prenatal Development

In 1885 the poet Coleridge made a statement radical for his time: "Yes—the history of a man for the nine months preceding his birth would probably be far more interesting and contain events of greater moment, than all the three score and ten years that follow it" (p. 301). The accuracy of this statement is only now becoming apparent. The months from conception to birth have an enormous influence on the rest of the individual's life: during the 38 weeks of prenatal development more growth and development occur than during any other comparable period of human life. The single fertilized egg cell becomes exceptionally complex as it increases its original weight more than a billion times during the period of only 266 days from conception to birth.

Three Changes in Viewpoint

Over the past two or three centuries Western beliefs about the various factors that influence a prenatal child have undergone three basic changes. An early view is that almost everything happening to the expectant mother influences her unborn child: the food the mother eats, her frightening experiences, the dreams she has, as well as things she sees. The philosopher Hegel (1894) contributed to this view with his theory that the mother and the fetus are an undivided "psychic unity."

Supporters of this view warned pregnant women that if a rabbit crossed the path in front of them, the baby would be born with a *hare*lip. Birthmarks were believed to be directly transmitted to the child as a product of the mother's experiences. For example, it could be dangerous to squash a strawberry during pregnancy, since the juices could be somehow transmitted to the baby who would be born with a "strawberry" mark. Maternal food cravings also could show up in the unborn child. Anatole France (1925) tells us:

Madame Morin informed the company that I had a red spot on the left hip due to a longing for cherries which had come upon my mother in Aunt Chausson's garden before I was born. Whereupon old Dr. Fournier, who had a great contempt for all such popular superstitions, remarked that it was lucky Madame Noziere had kept her desires within such limits during the period of gestation [prenatal development], since, if she had allowed herself to hanker after feathers, trinkets, a cashmere shawl, a coach and four, a town-house, a country mansion, and a park, there wouldn't have been enough skin on my poor body to hold the record of such inordinate ambitions. [pp. 11–12]

Such superstitious beliefs are clearly fallacious, but many hang on in popular folklore. Morrison (1920) describes the fears of a mother who had five healthy and normal children, and who had two teeth pulled during her sixth pregnancy. She believed that the removal of her teeth would somehow interfere with the development of her baby's mouth, and she became obsessed with the fear that her child would be born with a harelip. When the child was born with this condition, it was almost impossible to convince the mother that the extraction of her teeth was not the cause of her baby's defect. What appears as only an unusual coincidence to a scientist may seem like a causal connection to those who are emotionally involved in the situation.

If one were to believe that all aspects of the expectant mother's life directly affect her baby, the birth of a defective child could be blamed on the mother for some thought, vision, or experience she had during pregnancy. In one sad case a mother in her seventies lived with her fifty-year-old son, who had been afflicted with cerebral palsy since birth. This mother still regretted a train ride she had taken fifty years before during her pregnancy, because she believed that the jerky movements of the train were somehow transmitted to the son and caused cerebral palsy. She was tormenting herself needlessly. The only scientific evidence existing for any kind of maternal influence of this type deals with the mother's emotional state as affected by her environmental conditions.

Evidence disputing this older superstitious view has come through increased knowledge about prenatal development. It is now known that there is no direct connection between the mother's thoughts and fears and her fetus prenatally. So also are the physical connections between mother and fetus insulated from one another. Their blood systems are separate and do not mingle. Substances such as oxygen, water, and nutrients from the mother's bloodstream are absorbed into the baby's bloodstream though the placenta, which is attached to the wall of the mother's uterus and connected to the baby's body by the umbilical cord. Nor are there any direct nerve connections between mother and child. Because there are no nerves in the umbilical cord it would be impossible for the mother's thoughts, experiences, feelings, and emotions to have a direct influence on the unborn child.

Further evidence exists that disproves the superstitious viewpoint in that many of the same types of abnormalities attributed by traditional belief to maternal impressions are found also in the lower animals. But from what is known about these animals their low level of mental development would presumably make them incapable of such maternal impressions.

Another group of researchers held that nutrition was the only prenatal influence on the unborn child—that only through the food she ate, did the mother have any influence on the child she was carrying.

But such events as the thalidomide tragedy of the early 1960s, the rash of birth defects that followed the German measles epidemic of 1963–1965, and the new knowledge that even methadone (which is used as a substitute for heroin in drug addict treatment) can be an addictive drug for babies born to mothers using methadone have provided further evidence that there are many ways in which the unborn baby can be affected by its mother other than just through the food she eats. The mother's emotional state, her age, her blood type, the drugs she takes, the diseases she has, and the general state of her health are just some of the important influences on her unborn baby's environment.

Three Stages of Prenatal Development

Before discussing the specific prenatal influences on the unborn child, it is necessary to provide some background on the three prenatal stages of development.[1] First is the *germinal stage,* which is the period from fertilization until the end of the second week after conception. This period ends when the fertilized ovum, or technically the blastocyst (which is the term given to the hollow ball of cells present during the second week after conception), is implanted in the wall of the uterus. However, the developing organism actually begins to embed itself in the uterine lining some-time during the second week after conception (according to Tanner [1970] implantation occurs about seven days after conception). Thus the actual germinal period may be some-what shorter than two weeks. Second is the *embryonic stage* (from embryo, a Greek word meaning to swell), which is the six-week period from the end of the second week until the end of the second month after conception. By the end of this stage, when the first bone cell is laid down, the embryo has all the essential human parts and looks to a practiced eye like a miniature human being. The third and final stage, the *fetal stage* (from fetus, a Latin word mean-ing young one) lasts from the end of the second month until birth.

Germinal Stage

The germinal stage begins with fertilization, which occurs when one of the millions of sperm released by the male during sexual intercourse meets the ovum released by the female's ovary in one of the Fallopian tubes (see Figure 1 and Color Plate 1). The result is a fertilized zygote. (See Color Plate 2 for a diagram of the female reproductive sys-tem showing how conception occurs.) The 23 chromosomes

[1]The source for the following definitions of the three stages of prenatal development is Tanner (1970). Medical textbooks may provide somewhat different definitions of these terms.

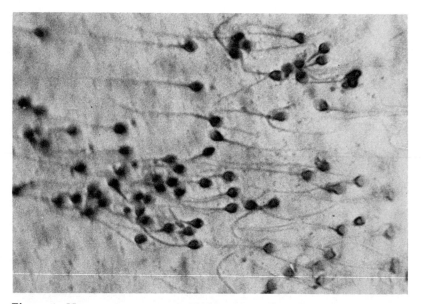

Figure 1. Human spermatozoa. Each sperm cell is about $1/500$ of an inch long. Millions of sperm are released in each act of sexual intercourse, but only one sperm is needed to fertilize the female ovum in order for pregnancy to occur. Courtesy of Dr. Roberts Rugh.

contributed by the reproductive cells of each of the parents align to form 23 pairs, and this arrangment is repeated in every one of the new individual's cells. These chromosomes contain the new individual's genetic potential and determine many of the individual's characteristics such as eye color and general body shape. They are not, however, the sole determinant of the individual's development, as almost from the moment of conception the environment also begins to influence the course of development.

The one-cell fertilized zygote divides into two cells, the two cells become four, and the process continues as the zygote descends the Fallopian tube and floats in the uterus before embedding itself (see Color Plate 2). Before each cell divides, the 46 chromosomes duplicate themselves. By about a week after conception a hollow cluster of more than 100 cells has been formed, and the cells have already begun to differentiate themselves according to their future functions. The zygote has now become a blastocyst (see Figure 2). At this point, two layers of cells are forming. The outer

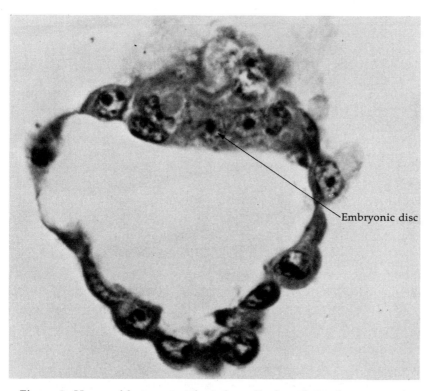

Embryonic disc

Figure 2. Human blastocyst at four days. By four days after conception the blastocyst has more cells clustered on one side than on the other. The cluster of cells labeled the embryonic disc is at this stage only two cells thick, but it will become the embryo itself. The purpose of the rest of the cells is to invade the uterine lining so that the blastocyst can attach itself and continue to grow and develop. Courtesy Carnegie Institution of Washington, Department of Embryology, Davis Division. Reprinted by permission.

21

layer serves the nourishing and protective functions. It will develop into the placenta, by which the baby is attached to the mother, the umbilical cord (which is the baby's lifeline for bringing in food and oxygen, and for discharging waste material), and the amniotic sac (the membrane filled with amniotic salty fluid that completely surrounds the embryo by the end of the eighth week after conception and acts as a shock absorber). The inner cell cluster will become the embryo itself.

The placenta and umbilical cord, which begin developing during the germinal period, are essential to the physical processes of mother-infant functioning. The placenta, through the umbilical cord which contains two arteries and a vein, supplies the embryo with all its needs, carries off all its wastes, and also protects it from damage in a variety of ways. Through the placenta the vein brings in food, oxygen, and other chemical substances from the mother, while the arteries return waste material from the baby to the mother for her disposal. The placenta, which is a blood-filled spongy mass that grows in size with the baby and ultimately reaches a diameter of about eight inches (see Color Plate 3), has two separate sets of blood vessels: one set goes to and from the baby, through the umbilical cord, and the other goes to and from the mother, through arteries and veins supplying the placenta. These two vessel systems, maternal and fetal, lie side by side and are intermeshed, but they are totally separate from each other. Because the blood-vessel walls are premeable, a constant exchange of materials (the food, oxygen, and waste dissolved in the blood carried through the blood vessels) takes place through the walls. This very indirect process for supplying the baby's needs is necessary because the baby is a parasite on the mother's body. Ordinarily the body rejects foreign material, and it is still not known how the placenta is able to disarm the mother's immunological defenses so that her body will tolerate a foreign body in her system for nine months.

In addition to trading off oxygen for carbon dioxide and food for wastes, the placenta also keeps out bacteria and brings in antibodies so that the baby will have short-term immunity (lasting about six months) to the same diseases for which the mother has immunity. By the end of this time the baby will have gained enough strength and exposure to the world to begin building up its own immunities. But the placenta is not perfect; it cannot always screen out everything that is potentially dangerous: viruses such as German measles, for instance, and certain damaging drugs such as thalidomide are capable of passing through the placental barrier.

After birth the umbilical cord is cut, and the newborn child must make the dramatic adjustment of bringing in oxygen directly from the air through its own lungs, and of filtering out and secreting waste material through its own organs. Once the placenta's mammoth job is done, the uterus contracts and pushes the placenta out of the mother's body (the afterbirth).

During the approximately two weeks of the germinal period the fertilized egg is basically unchanged in size, as it is nourished only by its own yolk. At the end of this period the future baby is about the size of a period (.) or about $1/175$ of an inch long.[2] The germinal period ends and the embryonic period begins when the blastocyst embeds itself in the wall of the uterus. Figure 3 shows a twelve-day-old embryo embedded in its mother's uterus.

It is possible to wash blastocysts out of the Fallopian tube and implant them in the uteri of foster mothers. This

[2] All weights and measurements given in this discussion are approximate (measurements vary considerably from one study to another).

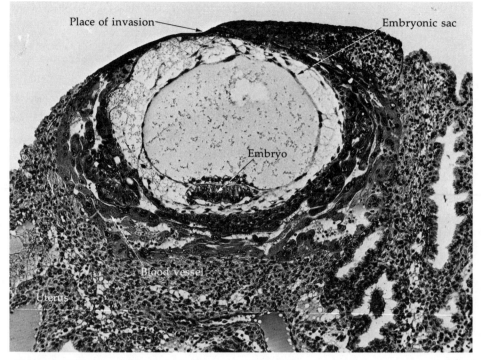

Figure 3. Human embryo at twelve days. This embryo in utero has been sectioned so that one may see how it has penetrated its mother's uterine tissues. The invading embryo destroys many uterine cells in order to penetrate deep into the uterus. Courtesy Carnegie Institution of Washington, Department of Embryology, Davis Division. Reprinted by permission.

process is already being done routinely in animals, in breeding stock (McLaren and Michie, 1956). For example, the blastocysts of larger Karakul sheep (from whose pelts Persian lamb coats are made) are conceived in Great Britain, where the breeding stock is located, and are transported to South African grazing lands in the uteri of smaller rabbits. On arrival in South Africa the blastocysts are returned to the uteri of other Karakul sheep. The benefit of this process is the savings in expensive air freight charges, and the blastocysts are not harmed by their frequent housing changes.

Similarly, scientists have experimented with the development of what are called test-tube babies (though it is the fertilized ova not the babies that develop in the tube) by attempting to fertilize human ova with sperm in the laboratory and implant the fertilized ovum in a woman's womb. One researcher reported a totally successful test-tube achievement, but then later denied it (Bevis, cited in Test-tube babies: now a reality?, 1974). Other researchers have reported the laboratory fertilization of a human ovum which they tried to develop to birth, since the ovum and the sperm that fertilized it were provided by a couple previously unable to conceive despite their wishes for a child (Wood and Lestong, cited in Human conception in test tube, 1973). But the fertilized ovum survived only nine days once it was implanted in the mother's womb. The first nonhuman primate baboon infant produced by blastocyst transfer from the mother in which it was conceived to a host mother was successfully delivered on September 5, 1975 (Kraemer, Moore, and Kramen, 1976).

It is no doubt only a matter of time until a human baby will develop successfully from test-tube fertilization to birth. The most important concern with such research seems to be the fear that blastocyst implants will result in abnormal offspring or lead to sacrificing the live child being grown in the test-tube: it has been predicted that test-tube fertilization of selected superior ova and sperm can eventually be used to weed genetically caused defects out of the human race. This possibility, of course, raises serious ethical and moral questions. Another possible use of this technique lies in helping women who had previously been unable to bear children.

Embryonic Stage

The embryonic or second prenatal stage of development begins once the blastocyst is embedded in the wall of the

25

uterus. After implantation occurs the embryo becomes a parasite, obtaining nourishment from the mother and discharging waste via the umbilical cord through the placenta, which develops adjacent to the uterus. Breathing movements begin in the fetus about the third month, but the fetus does not, of course, breathe the amniotic fluid, so there is no true lung breathing. For the time being, the exchange of oxygen and carbon dioxide between the bloodstreams of the mother and fetus occurs in the placenta. The embryo grows rapidly during this period, and by the end of the first eight weeks after conception 95 percent of the body parts have appeared through the process of differentiation, a process in which the formerly global mass of the blastocyst evolves into increasingly distinct and specific regions, such as the head, arms, and legs. Figure 4 shows a thirty-seven-day-old embryo in which body differentiation has not yet completely occurred.

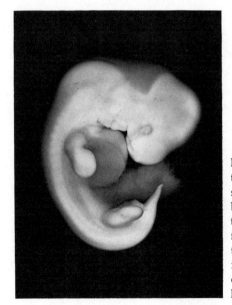

Figure 4. Human embryo at thirty-seven days. By thirty-seven days after conception the body parts of the embryo are in the midst of the process of differentiation. The tranquilizer thalidomide had its most damaging effects at this period of development. Courtesy of Dr. Roberts Rugh.

By the end of the first month three distinct cell layers have formed in the embryo (see Color Plate 2). From the ectoderm (or outer layer) the skin, sense organs, and nervous system will develop; from the mesoderm (or middle layer) the musculatory, circulatory, and excretory systems will develop; and from the endoderm (or inner layer) the digestive and glandular systems and the lungs will develop. The embryo is now only about ¼-inch long, but it is already 10,000 times larger than the original fertilized egg. It is crescent-shaped, with a definite tissue fold which contains swellings and markings that will become the facial features of the new individual. It has also a definite tail, but this soon becomes encased in the rest of the body. A U-shaped heart has developed and has begun to beat, so that blood flows through the microscopic veins and arteries. A primitive umbilical cord, a simple brain, and the early beginnings of the kidneys, the digestive tract, and the liver also exist.

By the end of the second month the embryo has attained a length of about 1¼ inches and weighs about $1/30$ of an ounce. Color Plate 4 shows a well-formed two-month-old embryo, along with its yolk, amniotic sac, placenta, and umbilical cord. At this stage almost all of the structures and systems found in a newborn have developed, and some are already functioning. Of course, these structures are very primitive and must develop further before they are considered to be completely functional. For example, a light touch to the mouth area of an embryo will cause the entire body to convulse, but spontaneous movement does not begin until later. The endocrine system (consisting of glands producing internal secretions) has begun to function; but while the male testes have begun to produce the male sex hormone, androgen, there are still no visible differences between the sexes.

The head of the embryo is clearly distinct from the rest of the body and takes up approximately one-half of the total body length. Thus in an 1¼-inch-long embryo the head area is over ½-inch long. The facial features of eyes, ears, nose, lips, and tongue are clearly present. Even the tooth buds are already formed. The forehead area is especially conspicuous due to the early development of the brain. According to the principle of cephalocaudal development, the sequence of human development is from top to bottom or from head to tail. Thus the head region is relatively large and complex early in life, whereas the tail area is small and simple. For example, the embryo's arms develop faster than the legs. As the child becomes older the increase in size and complexity of body parts proceeds downward through the body.

The first eight weeks after conception are a very active and crucial period of development. While the embryo by the end of this period resembles a miniature human being, an enormous amount of growth and development still lies ahead in the seven months before birth, but, basically, growth from here on will be an expansion of the bodily systems already present.

Since the development is so rapid during these first two months after conception, the unborn child is most vulnerable to many kinds of environmental insults and disruptions. Under a well-recognized developmental principle of critical periods, there are only certain limited times during the growth and development of an organism when it will react with the environment in a specific way. If the development does not occur at the optimum or critical period it may never occur at all, or it will occur with much more difficulty than if it had occurred at the critical period. Thus any serious environmental disruption during this first eight weeks can impair the whole developmental process, simply because another opportunity to complete the growth or correct the deformity may never occur.

For example, it is known that the first three months of pregnancy are critical for the development of the eyes, ears, and heart, and this is also the period when these organs are most vulnerable to the virus of German measles. On the average, one-third of the expectant mothers who have German measles during the first three months of pregnancy give birth to defective children. Deafness, eye defects, and heart disease are the most common kinds of resulting damage (Rhodes, 1961). Previously it was thought that brain defects and lowered intelligence also resulted from the effects of German measles during pregnancy. However, a subsequent study (Sheridan, 1964) found that while 30 percent of the 200 infants studied (whose mothers had rubella during the first sixteen weeks of pregnancy) suffered from various defects, their intelligence did not seem to be affected. The distribution of low, medium, and high intelligence among these 200 children was the same as among the general population.

Fetal Stage

By the beginning of the third month after conception the term fetus is given to the developing baby. The technical dividing point between the embryonic and fetal stages is the appearance of the first real bone cells that begin to replace the cartilage. Cartilage is the material making up the initial embryonic skeleton. (It is also the material from which the soft part of the adult nose is made.)

The private world of the fetus is a "warm, dark chamber, immersed in fluid, and provided by the placenta with continuous room service. It is protected from lights, blows and sounds" (Rodgers, 1969, p. 31). The baby in utero is an aquatic creature who has been described (Liley, 1967) as "a sort of combination astronaut and underwater swimmer. His movements to and fro, round and round, up and down have the wonderfully relaxed grace which we see in films of life under water. . . . He is really very busy, swimming around in his private space capsule" (pp. 25–26).

The fetal period lasts seven months and is the longest of the prenatal stages. The main events of this period include a substantial increase in fetal size along with an elaboration and growth of the bodily structures laid down during the embryonic stage. Because this is a period of seven months' duration and because so much growth and development is occurring, each of the seven months and its events will be discussed separately.

By the end of the third month the fetus is about three inches long and at long last weighs a full ounce. Color Plate 5 makes it possible to compare the size of a twelve-week-old fetus encased in its amniotic sac with the size of an adult hand. If removed from the mother's body a fetus of this age makes breathing movements and will make sucking movements in response to stimulation of the mouth area. The baby can kick, make a fist, and turn its head, but these movements are not yet usually felt by the mother. The eyelids are fused and will not open again until the sixth month. The fingers and toes are well formed, and the fingernails and toenails are growing. Because the skin of the fetus is so transparently thin the infant's fast-growing fingernails may put scratches on its face before it is born. Many babies are born already needing a manicure and pedicure.

Probably the most important and interesting event of the third month is the process of sex differentiation. The external genitals develop during this month, and the sex of the fetus can be determined by inspection. The development of the male sex organs proceeds rapidly, and for a time the female sex organs remain essentially neutral. In the case of the male, at about the ninth week, the action of the genes (a gene is a unit of a chromosome that gives one particular order in the construction of a human being) on the Y male sex chromosome (males have XY sex chromosomes) triggers a brief spurt of the male hormone androgen from the fetal sex glands or gonads, which causes the previously sexually undifferentiated gonad to become a recognizable testis. In the case of the female, there is no hormonal action since the female lacks the Y chromosome (females have XX sex chromosomes) and nothing happens during the ninth week, but at about the tenth week the gonad turns into an ovary. At about the fourteenth week the external genitals become female, and this too apparently requires no hormonal intervention.[3] If left hormonally alone, the fetus will always develop into a female.

During the fourth month the fetus grows more than during any other month. By the end of the month its length has doubled to six inches, and it weighs six ounces (see Color Plate 6). Growth of the lower part of the body has accelerated, and the head is now only one-third of the total body length.

The fetus has acquired a large repertoire of movements, such as sucking, turning the head, pushing with the limbs, the hands, and the feet. During this month the mother usually experiences what is known as the quickening, when she first feels the baby move inside her. At first the movements may feel like the flicker of a butterfly, but, as any mother will probably agree, the flickers become thumps by the end of the pregnancy. Moderate discomfort is frequent and normal during the later stages.

A fetus of this age can suck its thumb: Color Plate 7

[3] Tanner (1970: 114–115) in more detail discusses the process of sex differentiation.

shows a seventeen-week-old fetus that was caught in the act of sucking its thumb. Babies have even been born with callused thumbs from a large amount of prenatal thumb sucking. It has been facetiously said that mothers who are adverse to babies sucking their thumbs had best start their thumb-sucking prevention training early as their babies have a real prenatal head start on them. The prenatal practice of thumb sucking prepares the baby to suck spontaneously as soon as it is born.

The fifth month (or twenty weeks) is the midpoint of the pregnancy. The mother's condition is usually now obvious to other people. The baby is about twelve inches long and weighs about a pound. The fetus sleeps and wakes as a newborn does, and even has its favorite position in which to sleep. Babies born at this stage almost inevitably die quickly, since they are unable to sustain the necessary breathing movements.

During the sixth month the fetus adds another two inches in length and about a pound in weight. The previously fused eyelids open to reveal well-formed eyes. The red and wrinkled skin of the fetus resembles that of a very old person. Abundant taste buds have formed on the tongue and in the mouth. The fetus has a well-developed grasp reflex, can make slight but irregular breathing movements, and may even hiccup. A baby born at this time has a fair chance of surviving birth, but keeping it alive may require careful attention in a special nursery where oxygen is administered in monitored doses. The baby is capable of a thin crying noise if it is born at this time. Many cases of fetal crying in utero have been reported by doctors. In one case of a difficult delivery, where the fetal sac had to be ruptured to facilitate delivery, the crying of the still unborn fetus could be clearly heard by those who were attending the mother at her bedside (Graham, 1919).

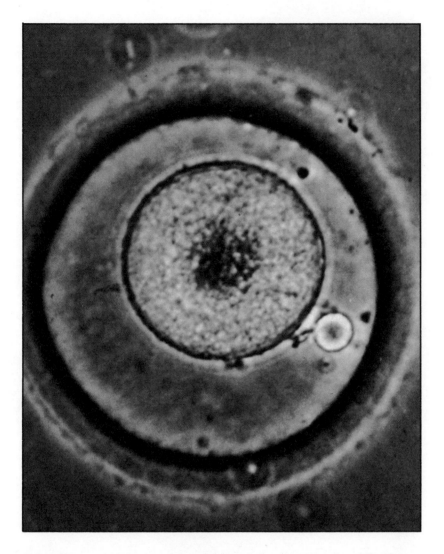

Color Plate 1. Human ovum. Approximately every twenty-eight days a sexually mature woman ovulates one ovum; it dies in about twelve to twenty-four hours if it is not fertilized by a sperm. The ovum is the largest cell in the human body and measures about $1/175$ of an inch in diameter. From R. Rugh and L. B. Shettles, *From Conception to Birth: the Drama of Life's Beginnings,* Harper & Row, 1971. With permission of Dr. Roberts Rugh.

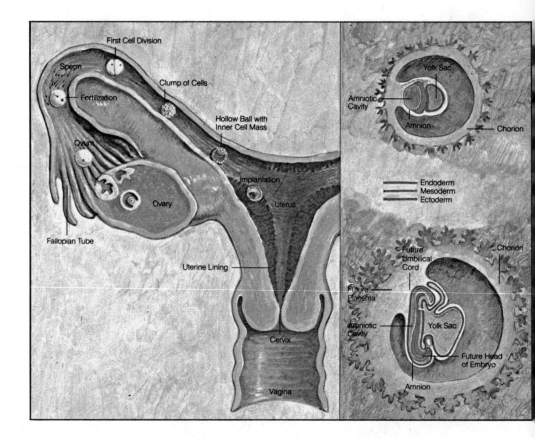

Color Plate 2. Early development of fertilized ovum and embryo. The sperm unites with th
ovum in the upper end of the Fallopian tube. The fertilized ovum divides many times as i
travels toward the uterus. The embryonic stage of development begins once the ovum i
implanted in the wall of the uterus. From *Developmental Psychology Today.* Copyright © 197
by CRM Books, a Division of Random House, Inc. Reprinted by permission.

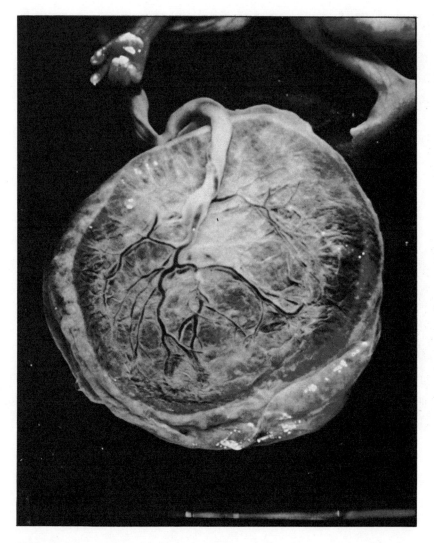

Color Plate 3. Human placenta at twenty weeks. By twenty weeks after conception the placenta covers about one-half the surface of the uterus, but it does not yet weigh ½ pound. Visible in this photograph are the arteries and vein through which the mother and fetus exchange dissolved nutrients and waste products. From R. Rugh and L. B. Shettles, *From Conception to Birth: the Drama of Life's Beginnings,* Harper & Row, 1971. With permission of Dr. Roberts Rugh.

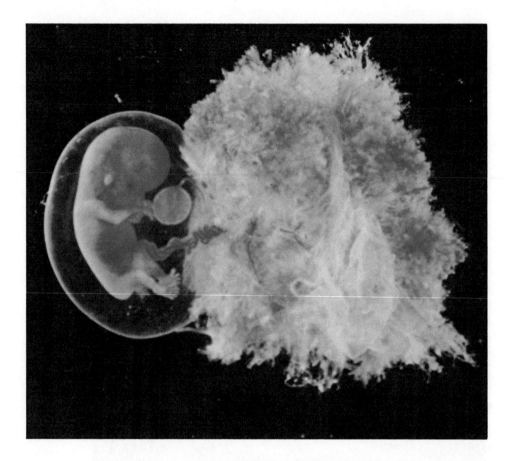

Color Plate 4. Human fetus at two months. Photograph shows a two-month-old fetus, together with its yolk sac, amniotic sac, umbilical cord, and placenta. From R. Rugh and L. B. Shettles, *From Conception to Birth: the Drama of Life's Beginnings,* Harper & Row, 1971. With permission of Dr. Roberts Rugh.

36

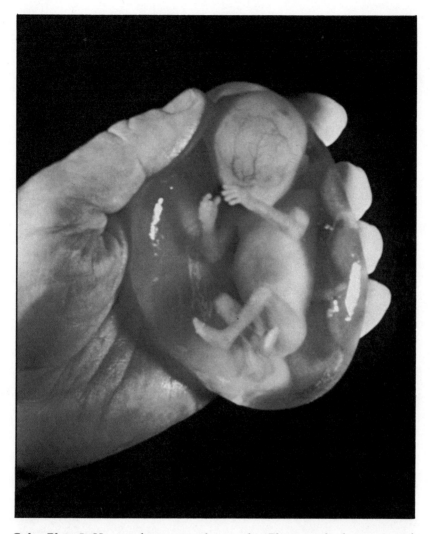

Color Plate 5. Human fetus at twelve weeks. Photograph shows size of fetus in relation to an adult human hand. When the twelve-week-old fetus is compared to the four-day-old blastocyst shown in Figure 2 or to a full-term baby at birth, it becomes apparent that growth and development during the prenatal period occur at a rate unmatched by growth at any other period of human life. From R. Rugh and L. B. Shettles, *From Conception to Birth: the Drama of Life's Beginnings,* Harper & Row, 1971. With permission of Dr. Roberts Rugh.

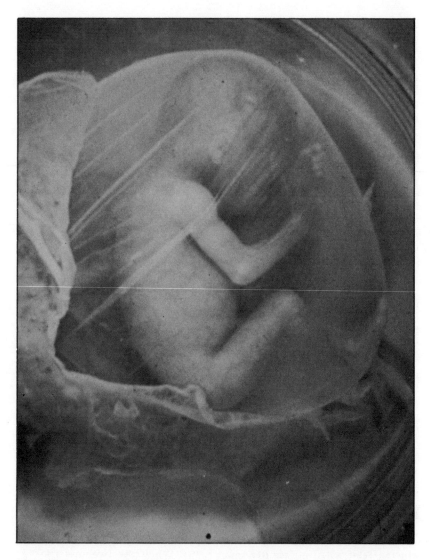

Color Plate 6. Human fetus at sixteen weeks. The fourth month is a period of rapid growth. The fetus gains about ¼ pound in weight and doubles its length to about six inches. This photograph illustrates the increasingly tight fit of the baby in its mother's uterus. From R. Rugh and L. B. Shettles, *From Conception to Birth: the Drama of Life's Beginnings,* Harper & Row, 1971. With permission of Dr. Roberts Rugh.

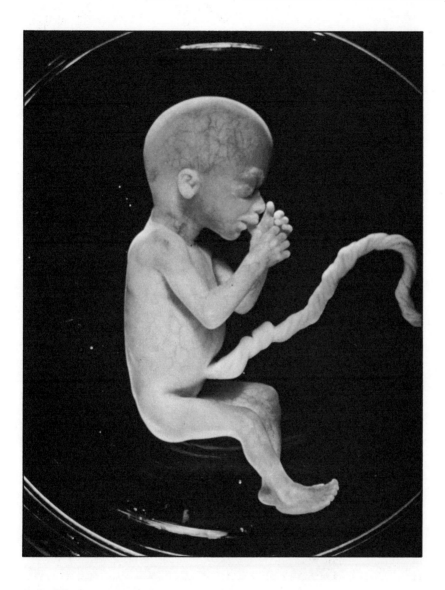

Color Plate 7. Human fetus at seventeen weeks sucking its thumb. Prenatal practice in sucking makes it possible for the fetus to begin sucking spontaneously to gain nourishment immediately after birth. From R. Rugh and L. B. Shettles, *From Conception to Birth: the Drama of Life's Beginnings*, Harper & Row, 1971. With permission of Dr. Roberts Rugh.

39

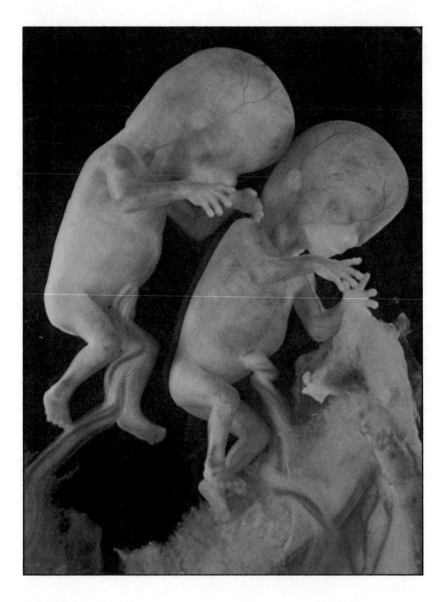

Color Plate 8. Fraternal twins in utero. This photograph shows the separate umbilical cords and placentae found in fraternal twins. From R. Rugh and L. B. Shettles, *From Conception to Birth: the Drama of Life's Beginnings*, Harper & Row, 1971. With permission of Dr. Roberts Rugh.

During the seventh month, which begins the last trimester of pregnancy, the growth of the fetus begins to slow down. It is fortunate that growth is slowed: it has been estimated (Rugh and Shettles, 1971) that if this did not occur, and growth continued at the rate of the first two trimesters of pregnancy, a baby would weigh 200 pounds by its first birthday.

At seven months (or twenty-eight weeks) the age of viability is reached, which means that the baby is capable of independent life and is likely to survive if born then. However, since the baby is highly vulnerable to infection, it needs a sheltered environment such as an incubator to survive. The incubator provides warmth and the short-term immunity to disease that the fetus acquires normally from the mother during the last trimester of pregnancy.

It is interesting to note, with regard to the need for a sheltered environment for babies born early, that the country doctor who delivered the premature Dionne quintuplets without regular medical facilities improvised incubators by placing each baby in a shoe box and putting all five of them in an oven turned to a very low temperature (Blatz, 1938). The five Dionne sisters were born in 1934 in Canada, and were the first recorded case of the survival of five identical children resulting from one birth.

During the eighth and ninth months of pregnancy the finishing touches are put on the developing fetus. The previously red, wrinkled skin rapidly fills out with fat as the baby gains about ½ pound a week. The action of the active baby is limited by the increasingly tight fit of the uterus.

The startle reflex is present; the baby responds to light and sound, lifts its head, and appears to be pleased when caressed. The effects of cephalocaudal developmental direction are seen again in that at birth the fetal head is 60 percent of its adult size. The brain of a full-term infant is one-fourth of the weight of the adult human brain, which still makes it relatively large for the size of the infant when compared to the infant's other organs that are about $1/20$ the size and weight of adult organs (Robinson and Tizard, 1966). The fetus has now reached full term, all intrauterine development has been completed, and the new human being is ready to live in a less protected environment than its mother's uterus.

At birth the average middle-class American baby boy weighs $7\frac{1}{2}$ pounds and is twenty inches long, while girls, generally, and babies from lower economic levels, are a little smaller in both height and weight. Despite its smaller size, however, the skeleton of a full-term baby girl at birth is approximately four weeks more mature (as measured by the amount of bone ossification—or laying down of real bone cells to replace the cartilage—that has occurred) than the skeleton of a full-term baby boy. This advanced female development continues—girls lose their baby teeth earlier and are thus visited by the tooth fairy earlier on the average than boys, and girls also reach sexual maturity on the average $1\frac{1}{2}$ to two years earlier than boys. The explanation for this phenomenon has not been definitely determined, but it is believed that it is the action of the genes on the Y male sex chromosome that slows the development of the male (Lovell, 1971). Females have an XX sex chromosome pattern and are not slowed down in their development by the presence of the Y sex chromosome which is found only in males.

The normal length of a pregnancy is 280 days from the beginning of the last menstrual period, or 266 days from the actual time of conception, but babies born from 180 to 334 days after conception have been known to survive. The prenatal period discussed in this book is the period lasting from fertilization until birth, and thus this time in the most extreme possible cases may vary by as much as 154 days (or over five months).

Multiple Births

The previous discussion has been concerned with the birth of singletons, which means that only one baby results from a pregnancy. However, a multiple birth is also possible where the arrival of two or more babies is separated by only minutes or hours. It has been estimated (Montagu, 1962) that the arrival of twins occurs in about one out of 87 births, of triplets in about one out of 7,569 births, of quadruplets in about one out of 658,507 births, of quintuplets in about one out of 57,289,761 births, and of sextuplets in approximately one out of 4,984,209,207 births. With the recent use of fertility drugs that often cause multiple ovulation, more multiple births of quintuplets and even sextuplets have been recorded, but chances for their survival are slim due to their unusually small size and the sometimes shorter period of prenatal development.[4]

Twins are the most frequent kind of multiple birth and are of two kinds. Identical or monozygotic twins come from the same fertilized egg, which, for some unexplained reason, later splits into two individuals. Siamese twins result if the separation of the zygote is not complete. Identical twins have the same combination of genes, are always of the same sex, share the same placenta, and are enclosed in the same amniotic sac although each has its own umbilical cord.

[4]The term "premature birth" is no longer considered correct scientific usage because the term does not provide enough information about the characteristics of an individual baby. This term has been discarded in favor of two more descriptive terms: low-birth-weight baby and short-gestation-period baby.

Nonidentical fraternal, or dizygotic, twins result from the fertilization of two separate ova released about the same time. It is believed that it is possible for either two ova to be released from the same ovary or for one ovum to be released from each ovary (Rugh and Shettles, 1971). Fraternal twins have separate placentae, amniotic sacs, and umbilical cords, and thus have entirely separate prenatal environments (see Color Plate 8). They are no more alike than two ordinary siblings. Fraternal twins may or may not be of the same sex; indeed, it is possible that they may not share the same father.

Identical twins must be of the same sex, while fraternal twins may be same-sexed or opposite-sexed. One mother had eighteen-month-old fraternal twins, Rebecca and Michael, who were of the same blonde-haired, blue-eyed coloring and of the exact same size. She was surprised at the number of people who would stop her on the street to admire her frilly-dressed daughter and pants-dressed son and inquire, "Are they identical?"

Triplets and babies born in multiple births of even larger numbers may be either identical if all come from the same fertilized ovum or separate siblings if each comes from its own fertilized ovum. It is also possible for any combination of identical twins and separate siblings to occur. It may be possible (Blatz, 1938) that in the case of the identical Dionne quintuplets one of the sisters developed from a group of cells which split off earlier than the other four. The umbilical cord for the five girls was a common one and branched for each embryo.

Several problems that are associated with the occurrence of multiple births center around the fact that two or more babies are crowded into the uterine space usually meant for one baby. They are thus more likely than singletons to die prenatally and to be born early due to inadequate space or nourishment. Especially in the case of identical twins sharing the same amniotic sac, the two may be unable to receive adequate nourishment from the jointly shared placenta. For example, it has been reported that two of the Dionne quintuplets who were smaller at birth may have been victims of an overcrowded uterus or an inadequate placenta. These two girls often turned blue from respiratory problems and were slower than their other three sisters in motor and intellectual development.

Montagu (1962) reports that it is beginning to appear that malformations occur more frequently among members of multiple births than among single births. Several researchers have reported that on the average twins appear to have lower intelligence than singletons. It is interesting to consider that in the whole recorded history of mankind members of a multiple birth have very rarely achieved fame and recognition.

The age of the mother also plays a part in the occurrence of dizygotic twins, as the chances of two-egg twinning increase with the age of the mother at least until age thirty-eight.

Another unusual variation of a multiple birth is called "fetus-in-fetu." This type of birth occurs maybe once in 100 million cases, and there are only ten or eleven such cases in recorded history, with only half of these being fully documented. The most recent case (Keating, 1973) was of a baby boy whose physician noticed a hard lump in his stomach during a routine six-week examination. X-rays of the baby's stomach revealed a spinal cord and the form of a fetus inside the boy's stomach. In the operation that followed, a fetus was removed from the baby's abdomen in much the same manner as a tumor would be removed. The fetus that was removed was not fully developed, but chromosomal tests showed that it was an identical male twin.

The baby who had the operation was normal in every way. This type of birth is called a monozygotic twinbirth, and medical science presently has no explanation for exactly how this occurs. It appears that the fetus starts out to be identical twins but that something goes wrong in the earliest stages of prenatal development.

2 Sensory Development and Prenatal Learning

Until recently it was commonly believed that the sensory environment of the newborn child was a mass of undifferentiated stimuli. In the famous words of James (1890), "The baby, assailed by eyes, ears, nose, skin, and entrails at once, feels it all as one great blooming, buzzing confusion" (p. 488). Research now makes it clear that the five basic senses—touch, taste, smell, hearing, vision—are operable in a newborn, although they are not as differentiated as they will be later in life. These senses develop during the prenatal period.[1]

It is well known that during the last months of pregnancy fetuses in utero respond with increased heart rate and bodily movement to loud and sudden noises such as the dropping of a metal pan or the vibration of a washing machine. One mother reported that attending concerts caused troublesome activity on the part of her eighth-month fetus.

An amusing story concerns a mathematics teacher whose baby was due two weeks after school was over in the

[1]Carmichael (1970: 447–563) provides a more technical and detailed discussion of the development of these five basic senses.

spring. She taught math to eighth graders who are normally quite interested in the origins of babies anyway.
They had been fascinated to watch the progression of her
pregnancy, and even went so far as to refer to her pregnancy as "our" pregnancy. One hot day in the spring
about a month before the baby was due she was standing
in front of her class going over the homework problems.
She was resting her book on her abdomen, which by then
protruded enough to provide a nice bookrest. All of her
students were at work on their homework papers, except
Rick, who was sitting at the back of the room. He happened to be looking at her when the pressure of the book
caused the baby to kick hard enough that the whole front
of her dress moved up and then settled back down. Rick's
eyes grew as big as saucers, and he stared but did not utter
a word to the rest of the class. However, by the time the
class returned to math the next day every student had been
advised of the amazing phenomenon they had missed the
previous day. The teacher reported she had never experienced such rapt attention as she received the rest of the
term, because all of them kept their eyes glued on her, determined not to miss the event should it occur again.

Touch

Before the layers of fat beneath the skin develop in the
last few weeks before birth, the skin of the fetus is quite
thin and wrinkled. It is also very red, because the circulatory system beneath the thin skin shows through. Most
studies indicate that the development of skin sensitivity
follows a cephalocaudal direction, beginning in the face
region and then progressing down over the surface of the
body. In animals this process continues on out to the end

of the tail. Pressure changes, temperature changes, whether hot or cold, and pain produce the skin sensations associated with touch.

The philosopher John Locke (1849 edition) maintained that a fetus is capable of sensing warmth. However, this is difficult to verify because of the constant-temperature conditions existing in the uterus. In studies of short-gestation-period babies (babies born early before completing the normal period of thirty-eight weeks of prenatal development or gestation), it has been found that by the age of viability at twenty-eight weeks their reactions to temperature are approximately those of a full-term baby. Short-gestation-period infants show responses to both warm and cool stimuli, with some studies indicating that their reactions to stimuli warmer than body temperature are stronger than to stimuli colder than body temperature. However, the temperature-regulating mechanism of short-gestation-period babies is inadequate, and necessitates the use of an incubator with constant temperatures.

Locke held also that a fetus could experience pain. Again, this does not seem to be totally verified by research. It is agreed that both the fetus and the neonate (a term for a baby during the first month after birth) show very little response to pain for several hours or days after birth. Sensitivity, increases rapidly, however, within the first few days after birth, as judged by the number of pin pricks needed to cause withdrawal of the stimulated area. There may also be constitutional differences among infants with respect to pain sensitivity, with females appearing to be more sensitive than males (Lipsitt and Levy, 1959).

In summary, research conducted on the prenatal development of skin sensitivity provides much evidence that the specialized skin senses are capable of functioning long before birth. Both the fetus and the neonate are capable of responding appropriately when a specific part of the body is touched or stimulated.

Taste

Taste buds begin to appear in the fetus during the third month, and by birth they are found on the tonsils, hard palate, and parts of the esophagus as well as on the tongue. By adult life, taste buds have receded to the tongue only, a condition which reduces the adult's potential for sensory stimulation from taste to less than the potential of the fetus. It is questionable, however, whether the fetus can use its apparently well-developed taste buds, because the composition and thus the taste of the salty amniotic fluid surrounding the developing child changes so little as the pregnancy advances that it is doubtful a taste sensation could be recognized. Even if taste sensations are possible, the fetus would soon become thoroughly accustomed to them. The taste receptors are well developed by late fetal life, though, and are ready to function after birth when taste stimulation becomes effective.

From experiments on the sense of taste done with babies born early at twenty-eight weeks after conception, and with neonates, it has been found that they react positively with a pleasant facial expression to sweet substances. While salt, sour, and bitter tastes give rise to unpleasant facial grimaces and a negative reaction, these three tastes are apparently distinguished from one another with greater difficulty and at a later age.

The human fetus in utero becomes capable of swallowing as early as the fifth month of development and normally begins to swallow small amounts of amniotic fluid. One obstetrician (reported in Montagu, 1962) took advantage of the ability of the fetus to swallow and its preference for sweet-tasting substances to treat expectant mothers suffering from an excess accumulation of fluid within the amniotic sac (a condition known as polyhydramnios). The obstetrician injected a small amount of saccharine directly through the abdominal wall into the amniotic sac. The fetus almost immediately started swallowing larger-than-usual amounts of the sweetened fluid, which was then absorbed through the intestine into the general circulation of the fetus. Eventually much of the fluid was returned as a waste product to the mother through the placenta and was excreted through her urinary tract. The very beneficial result was a reduction in the painful swelling of the pregnant woman's abdomen. It thus appears that the fetus is capable of discriminatory taste behavior, preferring the sweetened to the normally unsweetened amniotic fluid. It should be pointed out, however, that since the safety of saccharine has more recently been questioned, the use of this technique for reducing amniotic fluid is probably not very common.

Smell

Like the organs of taste, the organs of smell appear to be well developed early in fetal life. The olfactory parts of the brain are reported to be one of the earliest regions to be completely developed or myelinated (which is the process whereby a fatty substance that grows to cover the nerve fibers acts as a sheath and helps to speed up the transmission of nerve impulses). The question arises here whether it is possible for the fetus to actually "smell" substances when it is surrounded by the amniotic fluid. Again, the constancy of the composition of the amniotic fluid would appear to eliminate the changes necessary to produce stimulation of the sense of smell. It is probable that the normal kind of smelling does not occur until after the birth cry when the nose is filled with air. Infants born no more than one month early were able to smell substances, as evidenced by their turning away from unpleasant odors like ammonia and acetic acid.

Hearing

By late fetal life the hearing mechanism is well developed. The only structural change left to occur after birth is the draining away of the gelatinlike fluid filling the inner ear. This occurs within several hours after birth, or at least by the end of the first week after birth. It is believed that the fetus is probably deaf to sounds of normal intensity because of the liquid filling the inner ear. Many researchers, however, report changes in both the breathing level of the fetus and in its general level of bodily movements in the presence of a very loud noise, such as a shrill whistle or a loud automobile horn. In one of the earliest studies attempting to answer the question of whether an unborn child can hear, Peiper reports that one-third of the fetuses in his study responded to a very loud and shrill automobile horn with increased bodily movements.[2] Because the mothers were adequately prepared for the occurrence of the noise, he believed that the reactions were genuine responses of the fetuses rather than the surprised responses of the mothers.

Another famous example of apparent fetal hearing is the experiment conducted by Forbes and Forbes and reported by Carmichael (1970).

[2]The original report of this experiment by Peiper was published in German, but the study is also discussed in detail in English by Nash (1970: 277).

Thirty-one days before her baby was born a pregnant woman was lying in a metal bathtub full of warm water. A 2-year-old child was playing on the floor beside the tub. Accidentally the child struck the side of the tub with a small glass jar, and at once a sudden jump of the fetus was felt by the mother, which gave a sensation quite unlike the usual kicks or limb movements. A few days later an observer struck the side of the tub below the water line a quick rap with a small metallic object, meanwhile watching the mother's abdomen. A fraction of a second after the rap, a single quick rise of the anterior abdominal wall was clearly visible. The mother at this moment felt the same jump inside her abdomen as previously reported. Her own muscles were entirely relaxed, and she was not at all startled by the noise, nor was she conscious of perceiving any vibration through the skin. The mother's tactual sense later tested showed that the same intensity of vibration could be perceived only by those portions of the skin coming in contact with the tub. [p. 529]

Forbes and Forbes (1927) concluded with regard to their experiment that "good evidence exists that the human fetus 4 or 5 weeks before birth can respond with sudden movements to a loud sound originating outside the body of the mother. It seems probable that this is a true auditory-muscular reflex but the possibility of reception through tactile organs in the skin cannot be excluded" (p. 355).

A more recent study was also concerned with fetal hearing (Johansson, Wedenberg, and Westin, 1964). The reactions of fetal heart rhythms in thirty-two pregnant women were studied. Comparisons were made between fetal heart rhythms in infants exposed to tones of 100-decibel intensity for five seconds at 1,000 and 2,000 cycles per second. The mother's heart rate did not increase, but at 1,000 cycles per second the fetal heart rate accelerated by seven beats a minute, and at 2,000 cycles per second it increased by 11 beats per minute. Thus this study provides further evidence for the presence of fetal hearing and the ability to distinguish sounds.

53

Many researchers have speculated that because of all the sounds within the mother's body, such as intestinal digestive rumblings, rhythmic breathing, coughing, swallowing, talking, and the constant beating of the heart, as well as the loud external sounds to which the mother is exposed, the mother's womb must be a very noisy place. It has even been suggested (Liley, 1967) that if an expectant mother "should drink a glass of champagne or a bottle of beer, the sounds, to her unborn baby, would be something akin to rockets being shot off all around" (p. 31).

Salk (1962) has done a great deal of research on the prenatal significance of the maternal heartbeat. He feels the heartbeat is an important stimulus for the fetus, since the baby receives the steady beat from the heart as soon as its hearing apparatus has matured enough to hear. One of his experiments compared the behavior of an experimental group of neonates exposed continuously for the first few days of their lives to a recording of a rhythmic lub-dub heartbeat sound occurring seventy-two times per minute in a hospital nursery with the behavior of a control group of neonates in the usual quiet hospital nursery. The results showed definite behavioral differences—the experimental babies cried less, were more relaxed, fell asleep more quickly, and gained weight rather than lost weight as the control babies did on the same amount of food intake.

Other studies have found that continuous, rhythmic stimuli of many kinds, such as the tick of a metronome or the sound of a lullaby sung in a soft voice, are soothing to infants. One three-month-old infant was instantly soothed by the rhythmic running of an automobile engine and would fall asleep before the car was out of the driveway. The baby's parents joked that they felt secure in knowing that if all else failed in getting the baby to sleep they had a secret weapon—they could turn on the car engine. Salk points out that even adults find comfort in the rhythms of music. It may be that the calming powers of the human heartbeat are due only to the rhythmic and continuous properties found also in other stimuli.

Salk (1961) feels, however, that because of the infant's long prenatal experience in hearing and feeling the mother's heartbeat sound reigns supreme as a calming and comforting influence. The heartbeat sound is heard continuously in the early life of the baby, long before it experiences fear, and no doubt the rhythmic sounds gives assurance to the infant when facing some of the problems it experiences after birth. When an infant is distressed or disturbed and begins crying, the natural thing for the parent to do is to pick it up and hold it close to the chest—where it can once again hear a human heartbeat. Because the infant became accustomed prenatally to the stimulus of a human heartbeat, before it knew fear, it is now reassured and comforted by the stimulus to which it has been accustomed.

It has been suggested that evidence for the need to continue the calming effect of this rhythmical stimulus even after birth is provided by the preference shown by human mothers, as well as rhesus monkey mothers, for holding their babies on the left side. Dr. Salk (1973) observed a rhesus monkey whose newborn baby was held on its left side forty times and only twice on the right side, and often the baby monkey's ear was pressed against its mother's heart. Also in studying works of art from all parts of the world and all historical periods that depicted a woman holding an infant, Dr. Salk found that in about four out of five cases the infant is being held on the women's left side. This tendency is particularly noticeable in paintings of the Madonna and the Christ child.

In an observation of 255 human mothers and their neonates during their first four days after birth, approximately 80 percent of both right-handed and left-handed mothers held their babies on the left side. These findings led Salk (1973) to do a study comparing the habits of an experimental group of mothers, each of whom had experienced prolonged separation from her infant after birth for a period of at least twenty-four hours or more, with the habits of a control group of mothers who had handled their infants during the first twenty-four hours after birth. The control-group mothers showed a marked preference for holding their babies on the left side. Among the experimental-group mothers, those who had already had another infant with whom there had been early contact tended to hold the new baby on the left side, while the mothers of first-borns in the experimental group actually showed a preference for holding the infant on the right side. Salk concluded that the first twenty-four hours after birth is the critical period for the establishment of the left-side holding preference in mothers who, consciously or unconsciously, place the infant near the heart. Salk summarizes his findings in this way:

It is not in the nature of nature to provide living organisms with biological tendencies unless such tendencies have survival value. We often find in nature that the interaction between two organisms involves mutual satisfaction. In this connection when a baby is held on the mother's left side, not only does the baby receive soothing sensations from the mother's heartbeat but also the mother has the sensation of her heartbeat being reflected back from the baby. [p. 29]

Apparently mothers recognize, through a process of trial and error, that a baby is more easily soothed and quieted when held on the left side so that it can hear its mother's heartbeat. This heartbeat is connected with the uterine environment where the child experienced the greatest security it has ever known. In support of this theory a pediatrician (quoted in Montagu, 1964) reported that when she allowed her five-year-old son to listen to her heartbeat through a stethoscope he commented to her, "Mummy, I can hear your love flowing to me" (p. 178).

Salk's theory is most intriguing, but as yet his theory lacks further verification. It would be interesting to study the responses to a recorded human heartbeat among short-gestation-period babies who would have had less time in their mother's wombs to become prenatally imprinted to the maternal heartbeat.

Vision

The visual mechanisms are less well developed at birth than the auditory mechanisms, since major structural changes (such as differentiation of the visual part of the brain) are still left to occur in the visual apparatus after birth. Development of the cells essential to vision begins two or three weeks after conception. The eyelids fuse during the third month and open again during the sixth month. In the last six or more months before birth the eyes move with increasing coordination. During the last few months of pregnancy the eyes are apparently well enough developed structurally to make possible the light or iris reflex. A full-term infant is capable of visually following a slowly moving object, and is sensitive to patterns and contours within a few days after birth. Myelinization of the visual fibers is not completed, however, until about four months after birth; and improvement in the ability to fixate accurately and to see details (even though present to some degree as early as one week after birth) continues until about age six. The infant's eye is small and tends toward farsightedness: perfect 20/20 vision is not achieved until the child is about seven years of age.

Often the question is raised about fetal vision, since short-gestation-period babies are apparently capable of at least distinguishing between light and dark. According to Carmichael (1970):

There has been general agreement that the absence of radiation of the sort that typically activates the retina makes true sight all but impossible in prenatal life. The possibility does exist that under very strong light stimulation, if the head were in just the right place, radiation falling on the mother's abdomen might stimulate the fetal retina, but this seems most unlikely. [p. 530].

It thus appears that at birth the neonate is not at all an incompetent neophyte. In summary, the sensory abilities of infants do not differ markedly from those of adults.

Prenatal Learning

Only two studies dealing with the possibility of prenatal learning have been reported in the literature. Both studies were made in the 1940s and have never been repeated, but they seem to suggest that a fetus is capable of a very primitive kind of learning.

In the first study (Sontag and Newbery, 1940) the researchers made a loud noise near a pregnant woman's stomach. At first the sound produced a large change in fetal heart rate, but after the loud noise was repeated near the woman's stomach many times on successive days, the fetus no longer responded. Apparently the fetus had "learned" the sound, adapted to it, and thus no longer reacted to it.

In the second study dealing with prenatal learning, Spelt (1948) reported that he had conditioned the human fetus in its mother's uterus to give a startle response. In his experiment he paired a loud noise, to which the fetus would ordinarily make a startle response (unconditioned stimulus), with an electric doorbell with the gong removed so that it vibrated only. The doorbell caused no fetal response when originally applied to the mother's abdomen. However, after 15 to 20 paired trials with both the loud noise and the doorbell, the vibratory stimulus (or doorbell) alone elicited three or four successive startle responses and thus, in Spelt's terms, had become a conditioned stimulus. It appears, therefore, that the neural mechanisms of a fetus in the last months before birth have matured to a level in which learning (influenced by the environment) is possible. In other words, the fetus appears capable of acquiring certain habits of response while still in its mother's uterus.

These studies have been criticized for drawing very broad conclusions about prenatal learning from limited data. Also, it is reported that in the Spelt study there may have been inadequate controls on the mother's perception of the unconditioned and the conditioned stimulus which would have made it difficult to conclude that prenatal conditioning really occurred.[3]

It has been argued that short-gestation-period babies have an advantage in learning over full-term babies since they have spent less time in the isolated and unstimulating uterine environment and more time in the more stimulating outside world. This seems doubtful, and at present there is no research evidence supporting the view that a short gestation period is an advantage in learning, or in anything else for that matter.

[3]See Stevenson (1970: 854) for further criticism of these studies on prenatal learning.

Summary

The first two chapters of this book have been concerned with the internal development of the prenatal child, as well as with the normal physiological processes of mother-infant functioning. In normal prenatal development this internal development is to a large extent determined by the genetic information contained in the genes of each chromosome which have been inherited from the child's parents. According to Carmichael (1970), "the chromosomes with which each fertilized ovum starts life contain information for a set of enzymes that are in the genes of each chromosome. This is the 'blueprint' or 'coded punch card' that is the DNA, which as a totality constitutes the genetic code" (p. 451). Thus the prenatal child's internal development occurs along the lines dictated by its genetic code.

It is important to remember, however, that the developing child is an active system existing in an environment which also influences the child's development: the development of any human being always involves both genetic and environmental determinants. Thus, the developing systems of the child, which are directed by information contained in its genes, are also in constant interaction with the environment in which the child is developing. In line with this systems-interactive approach to prenatal development, the last four chapters of this book will be concerned with the effect on the unborn child of such external environmental influences as nutrition, drugs, and diseases.

3 Prenatal Effects of Nutrition

The "Self-Righting" Tendency of Prenatal Development

One of the most amazing characteristics of prenatal development is its "self-righting" tendency (Waddington, 1966). Despite the great variety and range of influences on prenatal development, there are a surprisingly small number of unfortunate developmental results. It has been pointed out (Sameroff, 1975) that

evolution appears to have built into the human organism regulative mechanisms to produce normal developmental outcomes under all but the most adverse of circumstances. . . . Any understanding of deviancies in outcome must be interpreted in the light of this self-righting and self-organizing tendency, which appears to move children toward normality in the face of pressure toward deviation. [p. 283]

The self-righting tendencies of the developmental process can be defeated in two ways (Sameroff, 1975). In the first instance, damage to the child's mechanisms for controlling internal development may prevent the functioning of the self-righting capability. This possibility is illustrated in children with Down's syndrome (Mongolism), who are born mentally retarded. An extra chromosome (trisomy), which has been consistently found in almost all individuals who show Down's syndrome, so alters the course of normal internal development that the self-righting tendency is unable to operate.

In the second instance undesirable environmental forces that exist throughout the pregnancy or at critical periods may prevent the normal internal development that would occur in a more ideal environment. An example of this can be seen in the damage caused by the German measles virus during the first three months (critical period) after conception.

When the child's vulnerability is increased through great damage to its mechanisms for control, only an extremely supportive environment can restore the normal growth process. Possibly the first successful example of restoring the prenatal environment to a more ideal situation for development occurred recently (Ampola, Mahoney, Nakamura, and Tanaka, 1975). In this case a woman had previously given birth to a baby that died three months after birth of an inherited disease called methylmalonic acidemia, a disease that is characterized by an abnormal buildup of acids in the body, continual vomiting, slow development, and failure to grow well. When the woman became pregnant again it was suspected that this second fetus might also be affected by the same disease.

When amniocentesis (the withdrawal of amniotic fluid surrounding the fetus so that the skin cells of the fetus and other substances in the fluid can be examined for abnormality) was performed, it was determined that this baby too was producing abnormal amounts of acids, an indication for the presence of methylmalonic acidemia. Amniocentesis also revealed that the cause was a defect of vitamin B_{12} synthesis: there was not enough vitamin B_{12} being synthesized to break down the amino acids in the baby's body. The mother was given large doses of the vitamin in the hope that it would pass through the placenta to help compensate for the deficiency in the fetus. When the mother began to excrete less of the methylmalonic acid in her urine (as a waste product from the fetus she was carrying), it appeared that the vitamin was reaching the baby. At birth the baby had only moderate amounts of acid in its blood and very high levels of the vitamin B_{12}. Apparently, the prenatally administered vitamin therapy had provided the supportive environment needed to help restore the normal growth process. At last report the child was three years old and growing normally, but it was still on a special diet to prevent an excess of the poisonous acids.

Nutrition and the Prenatal Child

While general public knowledge about the necessity for, and the crucial importance of, an adequate maternal diet during pregnancy has increased, many authorities in the field of prenatal development feel that inadequate nutrition still constitutes the greatest potential threat to optimum development of the unborn child. It is generally known that malnutrition during pregnancy is associated with a wide variety of pregnancy complications, among which are stillbirths, low-birth-weight babies (babies weighing under 5½ pounds or 2,500 grams after a normal period of prenatal development), short-gestation-period babies, and neonatal deaths, as well as many difficulties appearing in the offspring after birth, such as mental deficiency, rickets, cerebral palsy, epilepsy, speech defects, general physical weakness, and susceptibility to illness and disease.

It is not at all surprising that maternal nutrition so drastically affects fetal development, since the food supply for the fetus comes ultimately from the mother's blood through the semipermeable membrane of the placenta and the umbilical cord.

It is desirable for the woman to begin her pregnancy in a well-nourished state, for previous dietary deficiences are difficult to correct under the increased nutritional demands of pregnancy. A woman who enters her pregnancy with a good supply of an essential nutrient like calcium already in her bones will be far more likely to keep both herself and her baby adequately supplied than a mother who begins her pregnancy with a history of malnutrition. Even if the mother, prior to her pregnancy, is eating a diet based on adequate daily amounts of the Basic Four (meat, milk and dairy products, fruits and vegetables, bread and cereals) her caloric requirements will rise by about 20 percent during pregnancy, and her need for specific growth materials will rise even higher. For example, her need for protein and riboflavin increases by about 45 percent, and her need for calcium and ascorbic acid increases by about 100 percent above normal needs. The mother's diet must contain 2,000 or more calories of carefully selected foods in order to provide the protein, minerals, and vitamins required by both the mother and her fetus.

Nutrition is such an important prenatal influence that it even plays a part in determining the best time of the year for conception. Children conceived during the autumn and winter of the year are believed to have a definite advantage over children conceived during the spring and summer; investigators report that they are heavier, healthier, more likely to go to college and to be listed in *Who's Who in America*. It is reported, also, that mentally deficient children are more frequently conceived in the spring and summer than in the autumn and winter. In addition, pregnancy complications are more common among expectant mothers who conceived in the warmer months of the year.

One explanation for these findings is that women who conceive during the colders months of the year are likely to be eating heavier diets that include roasts, stews, fish, and eggs, which are excellent sources of the protein so necessary to the development of the child, especially during the first eight to twelve weeks of pregnancy when the brain is developing rapidly. Women who conceive during the hotter months of the year, however, are likely to skimp on these important sources of protein in favor of salads, fruits, and iced tea, and the effects may be detrimental for the developing child.

In another related study that demonstrates the importance of good nutrition for proper brain development, Knobloch and Pasamanick (1966) were concerned with the relationship between brain development and the season of the year when conception took place. Their subjects were retarded children and adults who had been born between 1913 and 1949, and who were resident patients at the Ohio State School in Columbus, Ohio. These researchers studied the connection between hot weather and the brain development of the babies, and reported that individuals who were in the first eight to twelve weeks of gestation during the hottest months of the year were most seriously deficient mentally. Their findings indicated that the hotter the summer, the larger the number of defective children that were born the following winter and spring. During the years with cooler summers there was no increase in the number of retarded born whose first eight to twelve weeks of prenatal development coincided with the summer and spring months. It seems likely that differences in the nutritional value of foods eaten by pregnant mothers during hotter and colder summers may partially explain these findings. It should, of course, be pointed out that the sample of patients from the Ohio State School studied by Knobloch and Pasamanick is not representative of the general population, but their study does point to the importance of good prenatal nutrition for proper brain development.

A group of studies by Dr. Joaquin Cravioto and his associates indicates that children experiencing early malnutrition both before and after birth perform less well on tests measuring such characteristics as physical ability and verbal ability in direct relation to the degree of retardation in height and weight for their age.[1] These studies were begun in 1958 in a town in Mexico where the social and economic differences among people were small. The town was chosen because the researchers were hoping to discover differences due primarily to nutrition. The data showed that deficits in height and weight at various ages were related to the individual's dietary history and experience with infectious diseases, and not to differences in personal hygiene, housing, proportion of income spent on food, parental education, or other indicators of social and economic status. Also, the performance of the children on intelligence tests and other psychological tests such as the Goodenough Draw-A-Man test was positively correlated with body weights and heights. Since all the children came from a population of relatively uniform socioeconomic backgrounds, Cravioto and his associates concluded that the most important factor causing shorter heights and weights in some children was poor nutrition during early life which also led to the lag in development of the skills tested by the psychological tests.

Many other studies have also shown that children born to mothers with good diets grow taller than children born

[1]See, for example, Cravioto, DeLicardie, and Birch (1966:319–372) for a discussion of this research.

to mothers with poor diets. This is no doubt the main explanation for American-born children of foreign immigrants being taller than their foreign-born parents (Greulich, 1958). For example, American-born children of Japanese descent are on the average about two inches taller than their Japanese-born parents. Dr. Merrill S. Read, Director of the Growth and Development Program of the National Institute of Child Health and Human Development aptly sums up these ideas:

I can't emphasize how important it is for the mother not to just trust that her body will somehow have the reserves that are needed for her infant. And a mother's nutritional reserves cannot be suddenly accumulated during pregnancy. These assets are the cumulative results of a lifetime. Getting ready to be a mother during a woman's adolescence is almost as important as the actual time when she's a mature woman and pregnant. It is particularly important before and during pregnancy to balance a diet with a variety of food from the four basic food groups. . . . Special attention should be given to foods rich in iron—liver, eggs, dark-green leafy vegetables. A woman should control her caloric intake by limiting fats and carbohydrates and make everything count nutritionally. [quoted in Wyden, 1971, pp. 93–95]

The Consequences of Malnutrition

The research on malnutrition makes it quite clear that extensive malnutrition, however defined, results in impaired physical development and lower levels of intellectual performance for the affected child.[2] Since one of the most critical periods for the growth of brain cells occurs prenatally, early malnutrition may cause irreversible damage.

Some of the data to be presented below on the effects of

[2] Vore (1973: 253–260) offers a good detailed summary of the effects of prenatal nutrition on intellectual development after birth.

specific kinds of malnutrition will be based on animal studies, for two reasons: first, because it would be unethical to experimentally manipulate human populations in order to create malnourished mothers and fetuses, and second, because studies using animals to demonstrate the effects of malnutrition are uncomplicated by the social and psychological factors so commonly associated with malnutrition in humans.

One of the early studies (Ebbs, Tisdall, and Scott, 1942) documenting the consequences of malnutrition during pregnancy was conducted at the clinic of the University of Toronto during the early 1940s. In this study 210 expectant mothers had eaten inadequate diets during the first four or five months of their pregnancies. The women were divided into two groups of 90 experimental mothers and 120 control mothers. The experimental group received dietary supplements so that they were eating nutritionally adequate diets during the last part of their pregnancies and for five weeks after their babies were born. The control group continued to eat nutritionally inadequate diets for the entire period of their pregnancies and for five weeks after their babies were born. The mothers in the experimental group, as compared to those in the control group, were in better health, had less toxemia (the cause of toxemia is unknown but the disorder occurs exclusively in human females during and immediately after pregnancy [Huffman, 1974]; less severe cases are characterized by high blood pressure, protein in the urine, and fluid retention while more severe cases are characterized by convulsions and coma superimposed on the above symptoms), less anemia, fewer spontaneous abortions (spontaneous loss of a fertilized ovum, embryo, or fetus without outside interference before it can survive outside its mother's body), and fewer stillbirths, short-gestation-period babies, and low-birth-weight babies. As an added extra bonus, their labors averaged five hours less in length. The babies born to the mothers in the experimental group were in better condition at birth, and they were healthier during their first six months of life, experiencing fewer serious diseases like pneumonia and rickets, and fewer colds and other minor illnesses.

The above systematic study shows the effects of good and bad maternal nutrition upon the course of pregnancy and the condition of the baby during the first six months of postnatal life. Much other evidence exists for the undesirable effects of poor maternal diet. In those countries suffering most from severe food shortages during World War II, the birth weights of live babies were reduced, and the incidence of stillbirths, low-birth-weight and short-gestation-period infants was greatly increased. In cases of extreme female malnutrition, such as occurred during the seige of Leningrad by the Germans, ovulation entirely ceased and conception became impossible. During the worst part of the Leningrad seige in 1942 under conditions of great food shortages, unheated homes in very cold weather, and the stresses of daily shellings, Antonov (1947) reported that for those mothers who did conceive 41 percent of the births were short-gestation-period babies. The mortality rate for full-term births was 9 percent, and among the short-gestation-period babies the mortality rate was 31 percent. These are all extremely high figures. Even the babies who were born at term showed the effects of the food shortage, as they weighed an average of twenty-one ounces less than the prewar average weight of newborns. In his study, Antonov attributed the high incidence of these problems to fetal nutritional deficiencies, and he minimized the effects of the stress and the extreme cold.

Additional research provides information as to which dietary deficiencies cause which specific defects in the fetus. Perhaps one of the clearest examples (reported in Montagu, 1964) of the relationship between maternal diet and its effect on fetal development came from Switzerland several decades ago. In some sections of Switzerland the soil contains almost no iodine, so the plants and animals of that area are also deficient in iodine. There was no natural way for the people to get enough iodine in their diets, and all were suffering from iodine deficiency. Pregnant women could not supply enough iodine to their fetuses to form properly functioning thyroid glands, and the result was the birth of a particularly large number of cretins, characterized by stunted and malformed bodies and slow mental development. After investigation into the problem by the government of Switzerland and the addition of supplementary iodine to the diets of pregnant women (as well as to the diets of the rest of the population), cretinism and its accompanying social and economic problems all but disappeared within one generation. This example shows quite clearly how disastrous nutritional deficiencies can be for the child, as well as how beneficial the act of supplementing the diet to reduce deficiencies can be in increasing the chances of normal, healthy development for the fetus.

Research with rats (Bronsted, 1955) has shown that if they were given a diet lacking Vitamin A early in pregnancy many abortions resulted, and that those young that lived suffered from malformations, especially of the eyes. By giving high doses of Vitamin A at certain stages of prenatal development, the occurrence of malformations could be reduced. The shortage of Vitamin B seems to be associated with lowered mental ability, and deficiencies of Vitamins D and C are associated with physical abnormalities such as deformities of the skeleton. Rat research has shown that, in general, vitamin deficiencies increase emotionalism and antisocial behavior while decreasing growth rates and the ability to learn mazes.

Excessive amounts of vitamins can also be harmful. Vitamin K assists in the clotting of blood and was at one time given to women and their neonates at the time of delivery to prevent internal bleeding. However, Vitamin K in excessive amounts is now known to cause damage to the central nervous system and mental retardation, so its use is no longer routinely recommended. Also, too much Vitamin D during pregnancy can result in excess calcium in the baby.

In other experiments, excessive amounts of Vitamin A given to rats during early pregnancy resulted in physical deformities, but if the large doses were given during later pregnancy the result was diminished motivation and attention span in the baby rats (Hutchings and Gibbon, 1971). Generalizing from these experiments with rats, it appears that a reasonable amount of all nutrients should be included in the human mother's diet in order to facilitate the growth of her baby.

Another study (Harrell, Woodyard, and Gates, 1955) points out that it is more difficult to establish scientific connections between *general* nutritional deficiencies and behavioral characteristics of the offspring than it is to identify the results of *specific* vitamin deficiencies and excesses. In this study to determine the effect of the mother's diet on the intelligence of her offspring, two groups of expectant women in both Virginia and Kentucky (four in all) were involved. The women in the experimental groups were given three different kinds of vitamin supplements until late in their pregnancy when they were reduced to only one of the three vitamin supplements. The women in the control groups received no vitamin supplements and continued to eat their regular diets. The results were interesting in that when the Virginia children were tested for intelligence at age three the children from the experimental group of mothers who had taken vitamins tested an average of four points higher than the children of the mothers in the control group. At age four the experimental-group children whose mothers had taken vitamins tested an average of five points higher. No significant difference was found between the three different vitamin supplements. However, in the Kentucky group no significant difference in intelligence was found between the children from the control and experimental groups.

The authors of this study attributed the apparently contradictory results to the different environments of the two groups. The Kentucky groups were basically well nourished prior to the study, because the mothers were isolated mountain dwellers who grew their own food and thus did not require vitamin supplements for their offspring. The Virginia groups, though, lived in a city slum environment, and the vitamin supplements had a beneficial effect on their offspring, due, it was believed, to the change from their previously deficient diets. This study, showing that maternal nutrition during pregnancy is capable of influencing the intelligence of the offspring until at least age four, is most interesting and has implications for the importance of proper prenatal nutrition.

Fallacies about Nutrition

A familiar saying is that "every baby costs its mother another tooth," meaning that due to the baby's demands on the mother's calcium reserves one of her teeth will be lost during her pregnancy and will have to be pulled. It is now known that with adequate nutrition and dental care this myth is absolutely untrue. It is correct that during the last three months of gestation the calcium requirements of the fetus increase greatly. If the maternal calcium intake is not great enough to meet the fetal demands, calcium will be withdrawn from the bones of the mother. However, there is no research support for maternal tooth decay or tooth loss resulting from this process.

Two other cherished beliefs have also been disproved by recent research, but they are still subscribed to by many people, and with potentially disastrous consequences for the developing unborn baby (Stone and Church, 1973). The first fallacy, now scientifically disproved, is that regardless of what the mother eats the baby has first call on nutritional supplies and will always get what it needs before she does. This view of the fetus as a "perfect parasite" was prevalent in many countries and, unfortunately, gave the mother complete freedom to eat any, and as many, nutritionally empty calories (for example, soft drinks, sweets, salty tidbits) as she wished, since—it was believed—the baby would get what it needed regardless. In line with this view, obstetricians were also recommending strict weight control during pregnancy. Some diet books even recommended pregnancy as the best time to go on a diet and actually lose weight.

This fallacious view presents an especially common problem among the large number of adolescent mothers found in the United States. During a recent twelve-month period 197,372 girls produced babies before completing their own physical growth, and 29,000 of these mothers were fifteen years of age or younger (Smart and Smart, 1972). A drastic example of the total lack of concern for adequate nutrition often found among such adolescent expectant mothers is that of an unmarried fifteen-year-old high school sophomore in her sixth month of pregnancy. She hated milk and never drank it. She had not yet told her parents about her pregnancy, and she had not been to a doctor for medical care. She was embarrassed about being pregnant and did not want to "show" her condition to other students, so she had gone on a rigorous crash diet to lose weight. At the end of six months of pregnancy not only had she not gained any weight, but she had actually lost fifteen pounds. The result of this pregnancy is not known to the author, but, based on the research discussed in this chapter, such severe maternal malnutrition during the period of gestation could be expected to result in offspring with deficits in body weight and maturation, fewer brain cells at birth and later in life, and later learning disabilities.

More is known today about the nutritional needs of both mother and baby and the order in which these needs are met: in the case of some nutrients, like vitamins C and B_{12} and iron, the baby will get its supply first, but in the case of other nutrients like vitamins A and E and iodine the mother's body has first call on the supply.

A drastic example taken from rat research shows what can happen to rats totally deprived of zinc during pregnancy (Hurley, 1968). Malformations such as missing limbs, brain abnormalities, curved spines, and cleft lip were found in 90 percent of their babies. Examination of the mothers' bodies revealed that they had adequate supplies of zinc in their bones and livers, but the fetuses could not withdraw it. Apparently zinc (at least in rats) is a nutrient upon which the mother's body has first call. Thus, the fetus must be supplied from the mother's diet during pregnancy rather than from her bodily reserves.

Another example of the baby's inability to get the nutrition it needs if the mother's diet is inadequate comes from a study (Holden, Man, and Jones, 1969) of eight-month-old babies of mothers with insufficient amounts of iodine in their blood during pregnancy. In all other aspects the pregnancies were normal. These babies, however, showed occurrences of cerebral palsy, visual and hearing loss, and mental deficiency, and scored significantly lower on tests of motor and mental ability than babies born to mothers with normal iodine levels during their pregnancies. Often babies are affected by the inadequate diets of their mothers and suffer increased chances of stillbirth, rickets, short gestation periods, low birth weights, anemia, and tuberculosis even though their mothers show no outward sign of malnourishment. In summary, if there is a nutritional deficiency during pregnancy, the unborn child may suffer, the mother may suffer, but it is even more likely that they both will suffer.

A second fallacy also totally lacking scientific support is the theory of "brain sparing," which holds that the brain is the last to suffer from nutritional deficiencies. Even if the brain eventually suffers from the malnutrition and slows down in development, it is believed that the brain will have a second, third, or even fourth chance to catch up, but this is most definitely not the case, for there are critical periods in brain development, and inadequate nutrition at those periods will permanently impair brain development with no chance to "catch up" later on.

There are four successive stages in brain development.[3] During the period of intrauterine brain growth, development centers on an increase in the number of brain cells (a process called hyperplasia): the brain grows bigger as the cells divide, and then divide again. Beginning at birth the brain enters a transition period where cells divide less rapidly, and growth of the existing cells begins. Around the child's first birthday the cells stop dividing, and all brain growth comes from an increase in cell size rather than an

[3]Dayton (1969: 213–217) has an extensive discussion of the four stages of brain development.

increase in number. The fourth and final stage is the formation of connections between the nerve cells, with every normal cell having around 10,000 connections. Some researchers believe that the number of connections between brain cells may turn out to be more important for an individual's intelligence than the actual number of cells possessed.

As noted in Chapter 1, the human brain is closer to its adult size at the beginning of the prenatal period than is any other organ of the body with the possible exception of the eye.

At birth [the brain] averages about 25% of its adult weight, at 6 months nearly 50%, at 2½ years about 75%, at 5 years 90%, and at 10 years 95%. This contrasts with the weight of the whole body, which at birth is about 5% of the young adult weight, and at 10 years about 50%. [Tanner, 1970, p. 119]

Nutrition has a direct effect on the growth of the brain, for without sufficient nourishment the rate of brain cell division will slow down. It has been estimated that a seriously nutritionally deprived fetus may have 20 percent fewer brain cells than the normal fetus, while malnourishment during the first six postnatal months can again slow down brain cell division by 20 percent. Thus, a combination of both intrauterine and postnatal malnourishment may result in a child with a brain as much as 60 percent smaller than normal.[4]

The relationship between brain growth and intelligence has been stated by Winick (1976) in this way:

Except under grossly pathologic conditions brain growth correlates with head circumference, and this correlation holds in nor-

[4]See Winick and Rosso (1969:774–778) or Winick (1976) for a more detailed discussion of the effects of malnutrition on brain development.

mal and malnourished children. The relation between head circumference and intelligence as measured by standard I.Q. tests adapted for various populations has also been studied. In affluent, well-nourished populations there is no correlation between head circumference and intelligence until the head circumference is reduced to such a magnitude that microcephaly [unnatural smallness of the head] is present and obvious brain pathology exists. In marked contrast, there is a high correlation between reduced head circumference and reduced intelligence in poor malnourished populations. [pp. 16–17]

Research makes it clear that the principle of critical periods applies to brain development, and that recovery will occur only if an improvement in nutrition takes place at a point in development when brain cell division is still occurring, that is, before the child's first birthday—when cell division stops regardless of whether the child has been well nourished or badly nourished.[5]

Animal research dealing with the formation of myelin also points to the falsity of the "brain-sparing" theory. Myelin, as stated earlier, is a fatty protection of the nerve fibers which helps to speed up the transmission of nerve impulses and reduces the random spread of these impulses. As the process of myelinization proceeds, both before and after birth, the animal becomes capable of more controlled movements and more control of the sensory functions. Research with animals makes it clear that myelin formation is impaired if the animal is malnourished during the period when the myelin is being formed. For the human fetus, the critical period of myelin formation begins by the sixth month of pregnancy. It has been theorized (Davison and Dobbing, 1966) that in human beings im-

---

[5]Bell (1974) provides an interesting account of the political problems that entangle any attempt to implement a government program to prevent prenatal malnutrition.

paired brain functioning and even retarded mental development may result from malnourishment of the mother during this critical period, with possibilities that are frightening to contemplate in view of the millions of babies being born to malnourished mothers all over the world. It points up the need for a worldwide program of cooperation to reduce widespread malnutrition, especially among pregnant women.

Winick (1976) summarizes the concept of a series of critical periods for brain development during which severe malnutrition will have maximum impact in this way:

Only during hyperplastic growth is brain cell number altered by malnutrition and only during the phase of rapid myelination is the deposition of myelin curtailed. Since these critical periods do not show flexible scheduling, not only is the brain particularly vulnerable during early development but deficits induced by malnutrition at this time cannot be made up later. Thus, a reduction in brain cell number due to curtailment of the rate of cell division by early malnutrition will not be corrected by providing adequate nutrition after the normal period for brain cell division has passed. It is from this kind of reasoning that the hypothesis of permanent structural and biochemical changes induced by early malnutrition has developed. [pp. v–vi]

Researchers feel that animal protein is essential to a balanced diet and proper brain development. Thus expectant mothers who are vegetarians will be nutritionally cheating their fetuses unless they are careful to substitute proper amounts of nuts, cereal grains, and beans for the meat, milk, cheese, and eggs found in the usual well-balanced diet. Expectant mothers on a macrobiotic diet that consists basically of brown rice may have such a large protein deficit that they will have difficulty carrying their babies to full term, while babies born live to mothers with any form of nutritional deficit are apt to have a low birth weight, and thus be less likely to survive the neonatal period.

Probably the most immediate result of the above findings has been to change medical thinking about the optimal weight gain during pregnancy. Many doctors have been limiting their pregnant patients to a weight gain of as little as ten to fourteen pounds. The Committee on Maternal Nutrition of the National Research Council recently alerted obstetricians to the possibility that this practice may be harmful both to the mother and to the developing fetus, and may be also a contributing factor to the high infant mortality rate in the United States. The Committee (quoted in Shank, 1970) recommended:

Weight gain in pregnancy should be closely monitored with the objective of achieving an average total weight gain of 24 pounds. This represents a gain of 1.5 to 3.0 pounds during the first trimester, followed by a gain of 0.8 pounds each week during the remainder of pregnancy. No scientific justification is found for routine limitations of weight gain to lesser amounts. [p. 11]

4 Maternal Characteristics and Experiences

The previous chapters have made it clear that the prenatal environment is different for every fetus and that there are many ways in which the course of fetal development and the later health and adjustment of the child can be affected. This chapter will be concerned with the influence on the developing child of such characteristics as the mother's emotional state, age, physical size, possible Rh incompatibility with the fetus, oxygen level in the bloodstream, state of fatigue, exposure to radiation, and personal habits in the use of alcohol, tobacco, and even coffee.

Emotional State

It is probable that almost all women experience some emotional distress during pregnancy, including some possible ambivalence toward the pregnancy itself. Whether pregnant or not, women continue to experience the joys, sorrows, and occasional tragedies of everyday life, but most babies are born healthy and normal because their mothers were able to deal with these emotional situations without harm either to themselves or to the development of the child within them. However, research with both animals and human beings makes it quite clear that *prolonged* strong and unpleasant emotional disturbances during pregnancy can result in behavioral changes in the child before and after birth.

Much of the knowledge regarding the influence of maternal emotions on fetal development results from the work done at the Fels Research Institute at Yellow Springs, Ohio, under the direction of Dr. Lester Sontag (1941, 1944, 1966). His studies with pregnant rats and other mammals indicate that severe and prolonged maternal stress, as well as crowded living conditions, can produce smaller offspring whose viability, activity and anxiety levels, and learning ability are affected. As early as World War II Sontag was writing about his fears that the emotional stresses of wartime bombings and anxiety about loved ones would affect the prenatal development of unborn children in Europe. He was concerned that these undesirable conditions would result in children born with functional disorders, particularly of the digestive system, or children who would exhibit unstable behavior patterns.

To say that an unborn child can be affected by the mother's emotional state is not a revival of the early notion discussed in Chapter 1 that maternal impressions influence the child's prenatal development. The blood systems of the mother and child are separate, but it is incorrect to assume that there is no connection between the nervous systems of the mother and child (Montagu, 1962). At times when the mother's emotions of fear, rage, or anxiety are strongly felt, certain chemicals are released into the maternal bloodstream by the nervous system, together with hormones secreted by the endocrine glands; and the metabolism of body cells is also changed. As a consequence, the composition of the blood changes, and new substances are transmitted across the placental barrier into the circulatory system of the fetus to create an abnormal hormonal balance. Thus, it is not maternal experiences and impressions that are transmitted to the fetus, but rather gross chemical changes.

The effect on the child of these chemical changes depends on the period of pregnancy in which they occur. Early in the pregnancy severe emotional stress can result in physical abnormalities. Harelips and cleft palates were once believed to be entirely hereditary. After studying a large number of mothers whose babies were born with harelip and cleft palate, Strean and Peer (1956) concluded that excessive maternal stress during the seventh to tenth weeks of prenatal development results in the release of glandular secretions that interrupt the formation of the fetal palate and the upper bones of the jaw which are forming during this period. Since about 25 percent of the mothers studied by Strean and Peer had cases of cleft palate and harelip in the family background, it was concluded by the researchers that probably both stress and genetic factors operate in the production of this deformity. There are, of course, other possibly incriminating factors, such as injected chemicals, drugs, and tranquilizers. In extreme cases of maternal stress the uterus can be affected to such a degree that early termination of the pregnancy occurs, perhaps with the birth of a fetus too immature to survive.

Stress later in the pregnancy is likely to result in behavioral changes in the fetus rather than in physical deformities. It is quite clear that the fetus is capable of moving in the womb; it hiccups and even sneezes as early as the fifth month, and its heartbeat can be clearly heard through the wall of its mother's abdomen. Sontag reports that when the mother is emotionally disturbed, the body movements of the fetus increase several hundred percent. The effects of brief maternal stress on fetal activity last for many hours, while longer periods of stress result in increased fetal movement. An extreme case of a prenatal reaction to emotional distress has been reported by Montagu (1964) in this way:

Possibly the earliest account of a connection between a mother's emotional state and a child's movements were recorded in 1867 by Dr. James Whitehead. He described a woman in her ninth month of pregnancy who nursed her twenty-month-old child, an only child, through a severe three-week attack of a serious disease. As soon as it was clear that the child would live the mother collapsed, exhausted. The child in her womb then began to kick so violently and for so prolonged a period that Dr. Whitehead called it a convulsion. The kicking grew more and more severe for several hours. Dr. Whitehead gave the mother chloroform and "repenthe" and the kicking began to subside. Twenty-one days after this, the baby was born, healthy and vigorous, and for as long as Dr. Whitehead observed him—a matter of thirty-five days—he showed no tendency toward unusual behavior.

Dr. Whitehead was well ahead of his time in his understanding of this episode. He pointed out in his report that although a child before birth may be quite unperturbed and unharmed by a physical shock such as [the mother's] falling from a height, "It seems to be otherwise when the mental system of the mother becomes unbalanced by violent and severe shocks of anguish, or by prolonged and severe anxiety." [p. 148]

Prenatal activity often results in low-birth-weight babies. Even when the birth lengths in inches are the same, prenatally active children do not weigh as much as less active fetuses because they have been employing a time-honored method of weight loss—increased exercise without increased food consumption. It is interesting to note that research at the Fels Institute has determined that active infants tend to be more advanced in motor development during the first year after birth than infants who were less active in the uterus.

83

After birth, the effects of maternal emotional disturbance show up in another way. Infants who are irritable, cry excessively, or have feeding difficulties are a familiar problem to both mothers and pediatricians. Sontag (1944) attributes such behavior patterns to emotional disturbance in the pregnant mother:

Another change which is apparent at birth in infants of mothers undergoing severe emotional stresses is in behavior, in total activity level. Such an infant is from the beginning a hyperactive, irritable, squirming, crying child who cries for his feeding every two to three hours instead of sleeping through his four-hour feeding. Because his irritability affects control of his gastro-intestinal tract, he empties his bowels at unusually frequent intervals, spits up half his feedings, and generally makes a nuisance of himself. He is to all intents and purposes a neurotic infant when born—the result of an unsatisfactory fetal environment. In this instance, he has not had to wait until childhood for a bad home situation or other cause to make him neurotic. It has been done for him before he has even seen the light of day. In certain instances of severely disturbed maternal emotions we have observed—for example, one in which the father became violently insane during his wife's pregnancy—the infant's bodily functions were so disturbed that a severe feeding problem resulted. The child was unable to retain food and became markedly emaciated and dehydrated. Experience with other similar cases suggests that many of the feeding problems pediatricians experience with young infants arise from an abnormal fetal environment. [p. 4]

In viewing the evidence regarding the tendency of emotionally upset mothers to give birth to cranky babies, it is important to point out that maternal stress most likely continues after the birth of the child; it is difficult, therefore, to separate the prenatal and postnatal causes for the behavior. Colicky babies, too, who cry excessively and who are apparently suffering from abdominal pain, have been born to mothers who were tense and anxious both during their pregnancies and after the birth of the baby. Again, it is difficult to separate cause from effect. Any mother is likely to become anxious if she is unable to comfort her continually crying child.

Age

The recommended time for childbearing is between the ages of 20 and 30 (Rugh and Shettles, 1971). The highest proportion of normal, healthy children are born during this period, which is also the time when the least number of complications of pregnancy such as spontaneous abortions, stillbirths, low-birth-weight and short-gestation-period babies, abnormalities, and maternal death occur.

The average woman's reproductive life spans the years from around 12 to 45 or 50. It is interesting to note that the earliest record of full reproductive capacity is that of a Lima, Peru, girl who in 1939 gave birth to a normal, healthy, six-pound baby boy when she was five years, eight months old. Statistics make it clear, however, that it is just as undesirable for a woman to have babies at an early age as it is to have them at a very late age.

Mothers under about 20 and over about 35 tend to have a greater proportion of defective children. These problems may result from an inadequately developed reproductive system in the younger mother, or from the progressive decline of the reproductive system in older mothers (Mussen, Conger, and Kagan, 1974; Pasamanick and Lilienfeld, 1955). The incidence of two-egg twinning that results in fraternal twins increases sharply to age 38, after which it drops rapidly. The occurrence of congenital hydrocephalus (water on the brain) is closely related to advanced maternal age. Mongoloids, or children suffering from Down's syndrome, are more common among older mothers. According to one authority, "The risk of mongolism is one in 3,000 for women under 30; one in 600 for those aged 30 to 34; one in 280 for those 35 to 39; one in 80 for ages 40 to 44; and one in 40 for ages 44 and up" (Apgar, quoted in Etzioni, 1973, p. 27). One study (Jalavisto, 1959) also found that the children of older mothers do not live as long as those of younger mothers.

Size

Shorter women, and especially those under five feet in height, are likely to have more difficult pregnancies and labors, smaller babies, and higher fetal mortality rates than taller women over five feet, five inches in height. Regardless of whether the women are short because of their genetic inheritance or because of environmental factors such as inadequate nutrition, they seem to be at a reproductive disadvantage in comparison to taller women. One of the major causes of difficulty seems to be the flattened pelvic brim, or edge, that is more commonly found in shorter women.

Obesity is another maternal characteristic that causes difficulty for both fetus and mother. One study (Matthews and derBrucke, 1938) of 200 women, each of whom weighed over 200 pounds, found that 75 percent of them developed complications of pregnancy, with toxemia the most common problem. (Toxemia is one of the most frequent causes of death in expectant mothers.) According to researchers, obese mothers also had more difficult deliveries, and their infants experienced higher-than-average mortality rates. Over half of the infants themselves were overweight, so apparently obesity is harmful to both mother and child. As a result of these problems, many doctors recommend that obese women postpone pregnancy until after a loss of weight.

Rh Factor Incompatibility

The word "Rh," as in Rh factor, comes from the first two letters of "rhesus" (all rhesus monkeys are Rh positive). In humans, the Rh-positive factor is an inherited, genetically dominant trait in the blood. About 85 percent of Caucasians are Rh-positive compared to approximately 93 percent of blacks and 99 percent of Mongoloids. The Rh factor becomes a problem *only* in the 12 percent of American marriages that pair an Rh-negative woman with an Rh-positive man (The unnecessary illness, 1973). Out of the 3.3 million births occurring in the United States each year, 260,000 result in the birth of an Rh-positive child to an Rh-negative woman. Approximately 10 percent of these 260,000 babies will be affected with some degree of Rh disease.

Laboratory tests can determine whether a person is Rh-positive or Rh-negative. For instance, the red blood corpuscles of an Rh-positive person contain a substance that clumps in response to a special serum (which has been prepared by injecting rhesus monkey blood into rabbits or guinea pigs). The blood of an Rh-negative person does not clump in response to this serum.

Rh disease occurs in the following way (see Figure 5). During the course of its development the fetus produces Rh-positive substances in its blood called antigens. The positive antigens are capable of passing through the placenta into the Rh-negative mother's bloodstream. The mother responds to the positive fetal antigens with the production of Rh antibodies. These antibodies pass back through the placenta into the fetal bloodstream and attack and destroy the red blood cells. The result is called

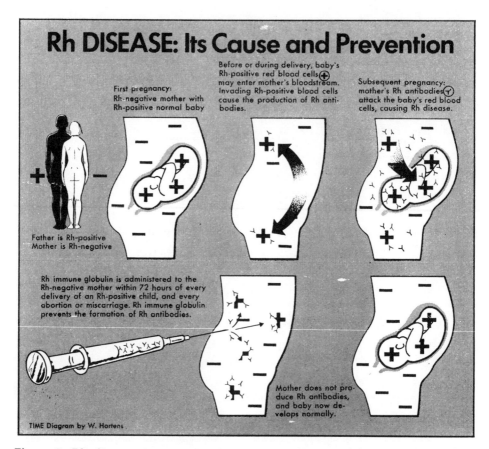

Figure 5. Rh disease: its cause and prevention. Reprinted by permission, from *Time*, The Weekly Newsmagazine, September 24, 1973; Copyright Time Inc.

erythroblastosis fetalis, a condition which leaves the fetus or baby severely anemic, due to the reduction in the number of red blood cells, and also jaundiced, since the toxic substances resulting from the destroyed red blood cells cause a yellowish cast to the skin. Depending on the severity of the problem, the baby may also be stillborn, brain damaged, or born too early to survive.

Even where incompatibility is known to exist, the first-born child is seldom afflicted, as the mother has not yet become adequately sensitized to the Rh-positive fetal antigens and her body is not yet responding with the appropriate Rh antibodies. In other cases the fetal antigens may fail to pass through the placenta, and, even if they do, for some unexplained reason the mother may still not respond to the fetal foreign antigens.

In the 10 percent of the cases where the baby is afflicted, there are now many ways to treat the problem. One method (the original treatment for Rh disease) is to totally replace the damaged blood supply with new blood by an exchange transfusion in which Rh-negative blood is used, so that the baby's life can be sustained until the maternal antibodies disappear from its circulation system. If the baby is being so seriously damaged prenatally that it will not survive until it can be delivered early, it is possible to use the Liley technique in which the baby receives an intrauterine blood transfusion before birth.[1] One woman who had lost 10 babies due to Rh incompatibility was successful in her eleventh pregnancy when the Liley technique was used. A method of prevention in use since 1968 is a vaccine in the form of a blood extract called Rh immune globulin.[2] This vaccine works only if the mother is not previously immune to the Rh factor. The globulin must be administered within seventy-two hours after a birth, an induced abortion, or a miscarriage occurring in any Rh-negative woman who is shown by tests to have been carrying (or who is assumed, as after abortions, to have been carrying) an Rh-positive child. The Rh immune globulin acts as a vaccine to stop the production of antibodies, and thus it greatly reduces the risk to future children carried by the woman. Used properly, the vaccine is nearly 99 percent effective.

[1] Liley (1963: 1107) offers a most interesting description of the development of this technique.
[2] Clarke (1968) discusses the development of this substance.

Since so much can be done medically if the Rh incompatibility of husband and wife is known in advance, blood tests for every expectant couple are now required by most if not all states. As a consequence of testing, and treatment with immune globulin when necessary, erythroblastosis is quite rare. It is also possible for an incompatibility in blood types to exist between mother and fetus, but the results are much less drastic than in Rh incompatibility.

Blood Oxygen Level

The fetus is totally dependent for its oxygen supply on the richness of oxygen in its mother's blood. Sensitive to a drop in the maternal oxygen supply, the fetus will squirm strongly in response to a threat of asphyxiation or anoxia. Anoxia occurs when the amount of available oxygen falls below the requirements of the organism. The nervous system and brain are extremely vulnerable to oxygen deprivation, which irreparably destroys nerve cells along with the functions they would have served. The damage resulting from anoxia ranges all the way from the death of the fetus by spontaneous abortion or stillbirth, to the less lethal but still serious damage of cerebral palsy, epilepsy, mental deficiency, and lowered intelligence, and a variety of behavioral problems of childhood including hyperactivity and difficulty in learning to read (Lilienfeld, Pasamanick, and Rogers, 1963).

Dependence on an adequate oxygen supply is highest during birth, at the time when excessive pressure on the head of the fetus (as it emerges from the mother's body) can cause hemorrhaging from rupturing of the blood vessels in the brain. Anoxia is also possible if there is a delay in the beginning of independent lung breathing when the umbilical cord is cut. Failure to establish independent respiration in this very critical period immediately after birth is one of the most common causes of neonatal death and of brain damage in surviving infants. However, a newborn infant has a much greater capacity to survive a shortage of oxygen undamaged than it would have later on, because the lowered body temperature at birth also lowers the bodily metabolism rate and thus reduces the requirements for oxygen. Many authorities are beginning to feel that the failure to begin respiration or to survive a period of anoxia may be due to pre-existing brain damage resulting from developmental or uterine causes rather than to the lack of oxygen itself. Short-gestation-period babies are especially susceptible to the danger of anoxia, for their bodies are not quite ready to begin functioning independently anyway, and they often have difficulty initiating breathing. It has also been suggested that anoxia may be a cause for the birth of short-gestation-period babies.

An unusual way to increase the amount of oxygen available to the fetus during the last three months of pregnancy as well as to reduce maternal labor pains has been developed by Heyns, a South African physician, and described by Denenberg (1967). Heyns designed a dome-shaped plastic bubble that is placed around the patient's abdomen. An air evacuation pump, controlled by the patient, is attached to the bubble, and can be used to lower the air pressure around the abdomen allowing the fetus to rise in the body cavity. The use of this decompression technique during labor has been found to reduce labor pains and shorten the length of labor.

Heyns believes abdominal decompression is also beneficial to the fetus, in that use of the bubble increases the available oxygen supply since babies do not normally receive enough oxygen for optimal development during the last trimester of pregnancy. Babies of mothers who experienced abdominal decompressions during the last three months of pregnancy had developmental test scores significantly higher than the babies of untreated mothers, with the highest scores found in those babies whose mothers had the greatest number of treatments.

Fatigue

Maternal fatigue may be related to anoxia. Some researchers believe that a possible reduction of efficiency in the circulation between the uterus and placenta and a resulting reduction of the oxygen supply might occur in fatigued mothers. Other researchers have looked for a connection between fetal activity and maternal fatigue, but so far no direct relationship has been found.

The question of exactly how much exercise and fatigue is desirable and exactly how much is detrimental for the fetus has not yet been answered. Many women work exceedingly hard during their pregnancies and still give birth to normal babies. However, obstetricians appear to agree that it is undesirable for the expectant mother to become overtired (Rugh and Shettles, 1971). Even though it is possible for the mother to recover from fatigue by resting, maternal fatigue causes hyperactivity in the fetus and also exposes the fetus to possibly toxic breakdown products.

Exposure to Radiation

As early as 1929 Murphy reported that exposure to small amounts of radiation in the maternal pelvic region does not appear to damage the fetus, but that large doses during pregnancy can result in physical and mental abnormalities in the offspring. He reported that in a series of 74 recorded cases of therapeutic maternal radiation, 51 percent of the offspring were abnormal, and that the most common defect was infants born with heads of abnormally small size. Regardless of these early findings many doctors continued to expose their pregnant patients to both diagnostic and therapeutic X-rays. But after atomic bombs were dropped on Japan in 1945 it was learned that the resulting radioactive fallout had done extensive damage to healthy human tissue. As a result, attention was at last focused on the dangers of X-rays. Neel (1953) reported a great increase in the number of stillborns, miscarriages or spontaneous abortions, and deformities among infants born to mothers who had been in Nagasaki and Hiroshima at the time of the atomic attacks. Central nervous system defects were very common among those whose exposure was within 1,200 meters of the center of the explosion. Within this radius, seven of the eleven infants that survived had microcephaly and mental retardation. (Microcephaly, however, which is characterized by an unnaturally small head size and severe mental retardation, can also result from a very rare recessive gene.)

The fetus is detrimentally affected by radiation in several possible ways (Montagu, 1962). Particularly during the first few months of pregnancy, massive exposure to radiation can cause death of the unborn child in the uterus. Even very low doses of radiation can cause malformations and, possibly, delayed malignancies and leukemia later in life. The fetus can be made permanently sterile. Radiation can cause permanent changes in the germ or reproductive cells of the fetus due to chromosomal fragments breaking away from the nuclei, and these mutations, 99 percent of which are harmful, could be passed on to future generations. The damage done to an individual fetus would depend on such factors as the dosage and its timing during pregnancy, as well as individual genetic tendencies, but the research

93

findings are clear-cut in demonstrating the grave dangers of exposure to radiation during prenatal development.

Smoking

James I of England was one of the first to criticize the habit of smoking, when he described it as "a custom loathesome to the eye, hateful to the nose, harmful to the brain, dangerous to the lungs, and in the black stinking fume thereof, nearest resembling the horrible Stygian smoke of the pit that is bottomless" (cited in Montagu, 1962, p. 360). King James was way ahead of his time in his awareness of the dangers of smoking as confirmed in the 1964 report of the United States Surgeon General's Advisory Committee on Smoking and Health. Other recent research has centered on the prenatal effects of maternal smoking. Evidence has been building (Surgeon General, 1971) from both human and animal research over the past forty years that cigarette smoking during pregnancy can cause low-birth-weight babies, spontaneous abortions, stillbirths, and neonatal death.

As early as 1935 Sontag and Wallace reported that the smoking of only one cigarette during the last two months of pregnancy produced a sudden speeding up or slowing down of the fetal heart rate. Smoking also can affect the whole circulatory system of the fetus. It makes no difference whether the tobacco smoke is inhaled, for its poisonous elements (such as nicotine and carbon monoxide) are still absorbed into the body through the mouth and throat (Smoking, carbon monoxide, and the fetus, 1972).

In a study of 7,449 pregnant patients Simpson (1957) found that heavy smokers were more than twice as likely to have low-birth-weight babies as were nonsmoking mothers. Women who smoked heavily had even lower-birth-weight babies than women who smoked moderately. A later study (Frazier, Davis, Goldstein, and Goldberg, 1961) followed up Simpson's work with a study of 2,736 pregnant black women and again found a significant association between low-birth-weight babies and smoking. The babies of mothers who smoked a pack or more a day had a low-birth-weight rate double that of nonsmokers. Also, infants of smokers weighed less than infants of nonsmokers regardless of the length of the pregnancy—an important point, because low-birth-weight babies are more likely to die within one month after birth than are heavier babies. Smoking, it is believed, may affect the actual mechanisms of fetal development rather than be the cause of an early beginning of labor.

The Frazier group felt these differences were due to three possible reasons. First, maternal appetite may be decreased when the mother smokes. Second, smoking may constrict the placental blood vessels and thus decrease the oxygen supply to the fetus. It seems reasonable to conclude that several constrictions daily for the length of time necessary to smoke a cigarette could interfere enough with the oxygen supply and growth of the fetus to reduce its birth weight. Third, it is possible that a woman smokes heavily during pregnancy for the same reasons (such as tension and anxiety) that also cause low-birth-weight babies.

On the slightly brighter side, evidence gathered from a massive study (Butler, Goldstein, and Ross, 1972) of almost 17,000 English pregnancies suggested that mothers who are lighter smokers or who give up smoking by the fourth month of pregnancy can reduce the risk to their babies. This study found that the effect of smoking is dose-related. The infants of heavy smokers (two or more packs a day) weigh less than the infants of light smokers (four or five cigarettes a day). Also, the infants of women who smoked throughout their entire pregnancy were of lower average birth weight than those babies born to mothers who smoked only during the first part of their pregnancy. However, both groups of infants (of long-term and short-term smokers) were smaller than the infants of nonsmokers.

Another study (Hardy and Mellits, 1972) investigated the possible long-term effects of maternal smoking on physical growth and intellectual development during the first seven years of life. For this study children of mothers who smoked substantially during pregnancy were matched with children of mothers who did not smoke. In agreement with previous studies, the babies of mothers who smoked were found to be retarded in intrauterine growth. At birth these babies were 250 grams lighter and shorter than babies born to nonsmokers, and they were still shorter at age one. By ages four and seven, however, there was no significant difference in physical size or intellectual ability. It thus appears that harmful long-term effects of smoking were not identified in children who survived the prenatal period and the first year after birth.

In contrast to these findings of Hardy and Mellits, the National Children's Bureau of Britain (cited in How mother's smoking affects her child, 1973) has now found that not only do the babies of women who smoke during pregnancy have a 30 percent greater chance of dying soon after birth than the babies of nonsmoking mothers, but they also report long-term effects. The Bureau found that the surviving children born to mothers who smoked were $3/10$ of an inch shorter, had poorer school adjustment, and were three months retarded in reading skills as compared to children born to nonsmokers.

The above discussion summarizes only a few of the many studies in which the conclusion is drawn that women who smoke give birth to smaller babies. One researcher (Yerushalmy, 1972) disagrees, because he feels that the birth of smaller babies is caused by certain behavioral and biological similarities found among mothers who smoke rather than by the effect of smoking cigarettes. In a study of 5,000 mothers, Yerushalmy found that smokers who gave birth to small babies also had other characteristics in common. For example, they had an extreme and carefree mode of life, they were more nervous and neurotic than the more relaxed and moderate nonsmokers, and they had begun to menstruate earlier. These findings are still tentative and not verified by other studies, but Yerushalmy feels that smokers represent a group of women whose reproductive experiences would have remained the same whether or not they smoked. He feels that the increased occurrence of low-birth-weight infants may be due to the *smoker* rather than to the *smoking*. His conclusions obviously warrant further investigation, but they are not supported at this time by other studies.

Research thus indicates that maternal smoking may retard fetal growth and may be associated with a higher frequency of low-birth-weight babies, spontaneous abortions, stillbirths, and neonatal deaths, as well as with possible long-term deficits in physical and intellectual development. More fetal distress, characterized by an abnormally high or low heart rate, is also found among children of smokers. Maternal smoking during pregnancy is definitely not good for either the mother or her fetus.[3] An increasing number of obstetricians recommend that their pregnant patients stop smoking, especially if they have a history of miscarriages or of giving birth to babies with low birth weight. Despite these disturbing findings

[3]Subak-Sharpe (1974) provides an interesting popular summary of the effects of smoking on pregnancy, as well as on infertility and sex performance.

and the recommendations of their doctors, some women still find that "the choice between a dessicated weed and a well cultivated seed seems often to be a quite difficult one" (Bernard, 1962, p. 43).

Alcoholic Beverages

A review of historical reports indicates that a relationship between chronic maternal alcoholism and faulty development of the unborn child was suspected as early as the time of the Greeks. For example, in the ancient city of Carthage a bride and groom were forbidden to drink wine on their wedding night in order to prevent the birth of a defective child (Haggard and Jellinek, 1942). It was not until 1973, however, that Jones and Smith reported finding a pattern of abnormal growth and development in their studies of eight children of chronic alcoholic mothers. Jones and Smith called this disorder the "fetal alcohol syndrome." The syndrome is characterized by defects that include prenatal and postnatal growth deficiency, microcephaly, abnormal develpment of the heart, defects of the joints, and facial abnormalities, especially of the eye.

A later report by these same researchers along with other investigators (Jones, Smith, Streissguth, and Myrianthopoulos, 1974) evaluated the records of a group of 23 offspring born to chronically alcoholic mothers. They found that 17 percent of the babies died soon after birth. The most frequent problems among the surviving babies were mild-to-moderate mental deficiency in 44 percent of the children, and abnormal physical features suggesting the fetal alcohol syndrome in 32 percent of the babies. A more recent report on the presence of fetal alcohol syndrome in 41 children (Hanson, Jones, and Smith, 1976) confirms the earlier results, but goes on to report an even more disturbing finding. Children affected with the fetal alcohol syndrome have continued postnatally to show slow physical growth in length, weight, and head circumference, as well as retarded developmental progress. Affected babies raised in good foster homes, in general, showed no better growth or performance than did the children raised by their chronically alcoholic mothers. Thus, the postnatal difficulties do not appear to be environmentally caused.

It has not been definitely determined what causes the fetal alcohol syndrome, but present evidence appears to indicate that the cause lies in the chronic alcoholism of the mother rather than in any possible malnutrition experienced by the mother. Hanson, Jones, and Smith (1976) hypothesize that since the prenatal growth deficiency for fetal alcohol syndrome children is greater for length than for weight, while infants who suffer from maternal malnutrition are usually underweight for length, then a factor other than maternal malnutrition apparently handicapped growth in the fetal alcohol syndrome children. These researchers believe that the undesirable effects on the unborn child are due to the direct effects of the alcohol (ethyl alcohol) rather than to any of its possible toxic breakdown substances or to malnutrition.

The potentially disastrous effects of maternal alcoholism appear clear. Now the question arises regarding the effects of moderate or social drinking. When the fetal alcohol syndrome was described in 1973, it was commonly believed that there was a cutoff point below which an expectant woman could drink without harming her child. A more recent study (Hanson, 1977) appears to disprove this belief. In a study of 74 moderate drinkers who consumed an average of two ounces of 100-proof alcohol each day both before and during their pregnancy, nine of their babies (or about 12 percent) showed one or more of the characteristics of the fetal alcohol syndrome. Abnormalities included small length and weight, microcephaly, a smaller than usual opening between upper and lower eyelids, and jitters and tremors. In constrast, only two of the babies born to a group of 90 mothers who drank little or no alcohol showed similar abnormalities.

Dr. Hanson (quoted in Henahan, 1977) summarized his findings by stating that

from our data we seem to be getting an early indication of a very crude dose-response curve relating total alcohol consumption to the outcome of pregnancy. Below an average of one ounce of absolute alcohol a day (two ounces of 100-proof whiskey), the risk for the obvious manifestations of abnormal growth and morphology [body differentiation] would appear to be low. In the range of one to two ounces of absolute alcohol (four drinks), the risk approaches 10%, while at heavier levels of five or more ounces (10 or more drinks), the risk could be as high as 50%. [p. 9]

Hanson's findings have been confirmed by Oulette (cited in Henahan, 1977), who found that for very heavily drinking mothers the risk of delivering an abnormal baby may be as high as 74 percent. The studies of Hanson and Oulette agree in indicating that even moderate drinking by the mother during the beginning stages of pregnancy can result in damage to her child.

Coffee

Coffee is another beverage now suspected of causing difficulties in prenatal development (Weathersbee, 1975). Among the women in the 550 families Weathersbee observed during 1974, he found that thirteen of the fourteen women who said they drank an average of more than six cups of coffee a day had an unfavorable pregnancy that resulted in miscarriage. He conceded that his study was retrospective and that he did not consider other factors which might have adversely affected reproduction. Weathersbee speculated that caffeine in the coffee is transmitted from the blood of the mother to the fetus. The increased caffeine levels in the amniotic fluid surrounding the unborn child apparently are associated with an increased incidence of miscarriage.

5 Drugs and Diseases

It has been known since at least the end of the seventeenth century that smallpox in an expectant mother could be transmitted to her prenatal child. In a large percentage of cases that child will be spontaneously aborted, but it is also true that the child may be born with disfiguring pock marks or even with smallpox blisters that show a still-active form of the disease. It is also possible for the fetus to acquire smallpox prenatally even though the mother herself is immune, if the mother is exposed to smallpox or is vaccinated against smallpox during her pregnancy. Vaccination during pregnancy does not increase the incidence of stillbirths, spontaneous abortions, or defects, but fetal infection with smallpox can occur. Unfortunately, there was a lag of three hundred years before anyone thought to apply the knowledge gained from experience with smallpox to the harmful effects on fetuses of German measles or rubella in 1941 and to the thalidomide tragedy of the early 1960s.

As discussed in Chapter 1, the old idea that the fetus is insulated from environmental effects by the placenta (which was supposed to prevent the passage of drugs and diseases to the child in the womb) is no longer scientifically supportable. The placenta prevents the passage of some harmful large-molecule materials, but it also acts as a passageway for many other substances, such as oxygen, drugs, gases, anesthetics, viruses, bacteria, hormones, and antibodies. The passage of antibodies can be favorable, as, for example, when the child receives passive immunity to many of the diseases (such as polio) to which its mother is immune—and immunity then lasts for several months after birth. The passage of antibodies can also be unfavorable as was seen in the discussion of the Rh factor in Chapter 4. The mechanism of the process, discussed earlier in Chapter 1, allows the molecules of the drugs, virus, or bacteria that are carried in the maternal bloodstream to pass through the placenta and the umbilical cord into the fetal circulation.

This chapter is concerned mainly with the teratogenic effects of drugs and diseases on normal fetal development rather than with abnormalities caused by defective and mutant genes. A teratogen is defined as any agent which produces or raises the incidence of malformation in a population; and teratology is sometimes called the science of monsters. Teratogens can be direct in their influence—as in the case of German measles which acts on the developing fetus. They also can be indirect—as in the case of a maternal thyroid deficiency which alters the mother's physiological state to the point that she is unable to supply enough iodine for the fetus to develop normal thyroid glands, and the child is therefore born defective.

The actual effect of a specific teratogen is dependent to a large extent on the effectiveness of the developmental principle of critical periods, which holds that there are certain definite periods in the growth and development of an organism when it will interact with a specific environment in a particular way which can be either beneficial or harmful. Generally speaking, the *stage* of development at which the drug is administered, or the disease occurs, is much more important in determining the extent and type of damage that will occur than the *strength* of the drug or disease. For example, mothers who took one tablet of thalidomide during the critical period of twenty-seven to forty days after conception were just as likely to have defective babies as those mothers who took many more tablets.

The effect of a drug or disease in the first trimester of pregnancy may be quite different from its effect during the last trimester. Much of the damage from drugs and diseases, however, occurs in the first two or three months of pregnancy, sometimes before the woman and her doctor are certain that she is pregnant. Indeed, severe damage can be done to the fertilized ovum or embryo prior to the end of the fourth week. This is because an interchange of toxic materials can take place in the fluids which circulate between the mother and her developing child before the placenta is fully functioning. The effect of a particular drug or disease on an individual developing fetus depends on many factors, such as the stage of development, the strength of the disease or drug, the part of the organism most susceptible to influence, as well as constitutional differences among individuals.

Drugs

It has often been asserted that the United States is a pill-popping society. Despite the fact that information about the many dangers of drugs is constantly increasing, the pregnant woman does not seem to see the danger. One California study (Peckham and King, 1963) found that the average pregnant woman takes more than three different drugs daily, and 4 percent of the women took ten or more different drugs. Because of statistics such as these, the National Foundation March of Dimes organization has mounted a major campaign to warn women of the dangers of taking any drugs at all during pregnancy. They emphasize in their public service announcements the importance of not taking drugs without the permission of a physician, who is expected to keep abreast of the properties of the drugs prescribed. This is not to say that all drugs are harmful. But, administered in the normal dosages, all drugs are capable of crossing the placental barrier, and a very large number of drugs are capable of affecting the fetus detrimentally.

The potential damage of drugs lies in two major areas (Montagu, 1962). First, the proper dose for a 125-pound mother will be a very large overdose for a one- or two-pound fetus. While the amount of the drug given the mother is not necessarily the same as the amount of the drug reaching the fetus, still, drugs are quite variable in their ability to be transferred to the fetus. Second, the fetal liver is incapable of breaking down the drugs in the same way as the maternal liver enzymes do, so the drug remains unchanged and acts on the fetus in a different way than it does on the mother. Newborn mammals do not begin developing liver enzymes until the first week after birth, and full development requires eight weeks. Apparently some factor in the uterine environment retards the development of liver enzymes.

Thalidomide

The thalidomide disaster provided a clear example of the effects of drugs on prenatal development. Thalidomide was never sold in the United States because of caution on the part of Dr. Francis Kelsey of the United States Food and Drug Administration, who did not feel that the drug had been sufficiently tested. But it was widely available in England, West Germany, and Scandinavia in the early 1960s and was recommended as an excellent nonbarbituate tranquilizer and sedative. Because it also helped to relieve the morning sickness typical of early pregnancy, it became a much sought-after medication. And, unfortunately, morning sickness was common during the critical period for causing detrimental effects.

Only fifteen cases of phocomelia (where the child is born lacking limbs, or with limbs in an embryonic stage of development) had occurred in West Germany from 1949 to 1959. But in 1960 several hundred cases appeared, and in 1961 ten times more cases than in 1960, so that a virtual epidemic of defective babies swept across the country. A frantic search was begun to locate the common factor occurring in the backgrounds of these defective babies. At one point it was believed that a chemical used in purifying the water supply might be the cause. By the time thalidomide was isolated as the common factor in all of the cases, 10,000 babies had been born with phocomelia. Approximately 5,000 of these babies are still living; 1,600 of them have artificial limbs, and many are also suffering from other malformations. So many thalidomide children are concentrated in certain areas of West Germany that specially equipped classrooms have been established to meet their needs.

When thalidomide was taken during the critical period of twenty-seven to forty days after conception, it interfered with the growth of the long bones of the arms and the legs, with the result that in the afflicted children the fetal hands appear almost directly below the shoulder (Taussig, 1962). The legs were similarly affected but with less distortion of growth. If the drug was taken after this critical period, the arms and legs were already permanently formed and there was no interference.

Other characteristics of the thalidomide syndrome include a temporary strawberry mark from the forehead down the nose and across the upper lip, a flattened nose in some cases, a missing external ear and downward displacement of the auditory canal (although there could still be normal hearing), paralysis of one side of the face, and malformations of the heart and circulatory system. Most of the afflicted children, however, have perfectly normal intelligence.

It is still not certain how thalidomide works, but it has been suggested (Montagu, 1964) that it chemically resembles another substance like a B vitamin or glutamic acid. The rapidly dividing cells mistake the identity of thalidomide and absorb it, but, instead of nourishing the cells, thalidomide stops cell division, concentrating most frequently on cells involved with growth of the long bones of the arms and the legs during their critical development period.

The whole thalidomide tragedy may be considered an unfortunate experiment in human teratology and development with but a single redeeming feature: by tracking down the exact day during pregnancy that the mother took the drug, and recording the particular deformities in her child, it has been possible to learn more about the schedule of prenatal development.

The Birth-Control Pill and Other Hormones Produced outside the Body

Evidence exists (Janerich, Piper, and Glebatis, 1974) linking hormones introduced into the body (such as birth-control pills) with limb malformations in offspring. This study matched (according to age and race) 108 mothers of babies born with part of a limb or an entire limb missing with 108 mothers of normal babies. It was found that 14 percent of the mothers with malformed children had been exposed to hormones during pregnancy, but only 4 percent of the mothers of normal babies had been similarly exposed. Exposure took one of three forms: unintentionally continuing to use birth-control pills after pregnancy had already occurred, using estrogen or progesterone hormones in the treatment of reproductive system disorders, or undergoing the kind of pregnancy test that requires the use of hormones.

In eleven of the fifteen cases of malformation the mothers received the hormones orally rather than through injection, and the affected babies were all boys. These results indicate that the use of orally administered hormones during pregnancy may have a sex-specific effect on the developing fetus. That is, they appear to cause abnormalities only in male babies. The Janerich group found also that the injection of hormones into four of the women resulted in both male and female malformed babies and they have tentatively suggested that these sex-specific effects result from the fact that oral hormones are chemically derived from the male hormone testosterone, while the injectable hormones are not. It is possible that the converted male hormone has a damaging effect on the developing child. These results are still preliminary, and more research is needed before a definite link is established between hormones and birth defects.[1]

[1]Janerich, Piper, and Glebatis (1974), as well as an editorial by Nora and Nora in the same issue of the medical journal, give more details on research linking hormones and birth defects. An interesting related finding that is discussed in the work of J. W. Money in Prenatal sex hormone levels: a possible link to intelligence (1972:8), suggests that a prenatal excess of the fetal sex hormone androgen, which is a male sex hormone, may result in increased intelligence.

Aspirin and Tranquilizers

According to research conducted by the federally sponsored Collaborative Perinatal Project, moderate use of aspirin during pregnancy appears to be safe (Zimmerman, 1976). This study compared the health records of 40,000 American women—aspirin users and nonaspirin users—and their babies and found no evidence that aspirin causes stillbirth, low birth weight, birth defects, or infant death.

These findings are in contrast to a smaller, earlier Australian study which found an increased risk of death in newborns whose mothers had used aspirin heavily every day during pregnancy. The findings of the Collaborative Perinatal Project discussed above are also somewhat in conflict with the tentative conclusions of a special panel of the Food and Drug Administration (Pregnant women warned against pain relievers, 1976). According to this panel, aspirin and similar pain relievers should not be used by women during the final three months of pregnancy except on the advice of a physician. The committee found that aspirin could prolong labor and lengthen clotting and bleeding times for both mother and baby.

The United States Food and Drug Administration has issued a warning that several popular tranquilizers may cause cleft palate and other birth defects if taken by a pregnant woman during the first months of prenatal development (Zimmerman, 1976). The manufacturers of these drugs dispute the evidence, but the Federal Drug Administration warns women in the first trimester of pregnancy to avoid taking any kind of tranquilizer. It is recommended that any potentially pregnant woman (a woman of childbearing age is potentially pregnant during any month in which she has engaged in sexual intercourse without adequate contraceptive protection; definition taken from

Drugs in pregnancy: are they safe?, 1967) should be very cautious in her use of drugs, since pregnancy may not be detected until very near the end of the first trimester.

Drugs prior to and during Delivery

According to the Bible, women should have "pain in childbearing and in pain you shall bring forth children" (Genesis 3:16). When anesthetics, such as alcohol and narcotics, began to be used in the nineteenth century many midwives objected on the grounds that their use was against the will of God. Today, a return to natural childbirth is advocated by some.[2] One of its advantages, it is claimed, is that the fully conscious mother can immediately start to know her child. Another advantage is the avoidance in the bloodstream of drugs which might prevent the vigorous breathing and crying so important in the first few days of life. Despite these potential advantages associated with natural childbirth, a study of almost 20,000 deliveries found that only 14.6 percent of the mothers received no anesthetic, and it was estimated that the number of those who, in addition, received no analgesic was quite small (Benson, Shubeck, Clark, Berendes, Weiss, and Deutschberger, 1965).

There is general agreement in the literature that the analgesics and anesthetics used in delivery pass through the placenta to enter the fetal bloodstream and fetal tissues within as little as one minute.[3] This passage of drugs into

[2] Bernard (1973:65–68) provides an enthusiastic personal account of the virtues of natural childbirth.

[3] Bowes, Brackbill, Conway, and Steinschneider, 1970, provide an authoritative summary of the effects of delivery medication on the fetus and infant as written by an obstetrician, two child psychologists, and a pediatrician.

the fetus is accompanied by a reduction of oxygen in the fetal bloodstream at least partially resulting from the reduced maternal blood pressure produced by the anesthesia. The potential neonatal depressant effect of analgesics and anesthetics has been described by Eastman (1959) in this way: "I am certain that any obstetrician of experience with sedative drugs would agree that the onset of respiration is usually less prompt and less vigorous when sedative drugs have been given than when they have been completely withheld" (p. 34).

The results of many studies make it clear that delivery medications can interfere with the immediate physiological adjustments required by the neonate to remain alive. It is also important to learn what, if any, are the long-term effects of delivery medication.

Stechler (1964), for example, found that the attentiveness of an experimental group of twenty full-term babies from two to four days old was affected if the mother had been given a depressant such as meperidine (Demerol) within 90 minutes of delivery, a period long enough for the drug to have reached its maximum potential in the fetus before delivery. When tested with a series of three pictures, each shown for one minute, the attention span of the experimental group of babies was shorter than that of the control group of babies whose mothers had received no drugs within 90 minutes of delivery. It was also noted that the more drugs that were administered (in amount of dosage and/or in number of drugs) and the closer to the time of delivery they were given, the less likely was the baby to be attentive to the pictures. The author points out that the question of the persistence of the effect of medication during labor on this kind of alert visual attentiveness beyond the age of four days has not yet been studied. But based on findings that drug influence persists longer in neonates than in adults, it is probable that an immature neonate has a susceptibility to the influence of drugs lasting longer than four days.

Another study (Conway and Brackbill, 1970) noted that anesthesia and analgesia have a definite effect on suppression of sensorimotor functions in the neonate. This study found that babies of mothers subjected to this kind of medication lagged significantly in muscular, visual, and neural development behind babies whose mothers were not medicated. Many of the difficulties ceased from two to five days after birth, but some effects remained until the baby was at least five months old. The researchers stress the need for more work in this area before definite conclusions are reached.

Many obstetricians feel, however, that it would be very callous to recommend the total withholding of drugs from women during even normal labor. These obstetricians feel that drugs for the relief of pain have a very proper use and can be safely given to most laboring mothers if proper attention is given to the type, amount, and method of administration of the drug. Drugs may, of course, also be necessary for delivery complications, as in the case of breech births (when the baby is born presenting its buttocks rather than its head at the opening of the birth canal). Despite the fact, however, that an estimated 85 percent (Benson, Shubeck, Clark, Berendes, Weiss, and Deutschberger, 1965) of all women receive medication during labor, the possibility that these "methods of pain relief may have untoward [unfavorable] consequences for both mother and infant must also be recognized" (Bowes, 1970, p. 13).

In summary of the effects of drugs administered prior to and during delivery, it has been stated (Becker and Donnell, 1952):

Volatile anesthetics and, especially, the barbituate derivates, which cross the placental barrier readily, can be every bit as effective in embarrassing the fetal respiratory system as our more direct methods of clamping the maternal uterine vessels. The warning to expectant mothers is obvious: It is not wise to insist on being "snowed under" at delivery. A little pain at childbirth, mollified [reduced] by light sedation, may prevent extreme sorrow later. [p. 161]

Drug Addiction

Heroin

Babies born to heroin-addicted mothers are usually smaller than average, with many weighing under 5½ pounds. It is not known whether this is due to the heroin, poor prenatal care, or perhaps even to a short gestation period. (Since the menstrual cycles of heroin addicts are very irregular, it is difficult to determine the exact time of conception.)

A large number of studies have reported a high incidence of maternal complications in addicted mothers such as toxemia, premature separation of placenta, retained placenta (rather than being naturally expelled as the afterbirth), hemorrhaging after birth, and breech deliveries. A high rate of neonatal disease and mortality has also been reported.

Several studies have indicated that babies born to mothers addicted to heroin are themselves addicted to the drug and must undergo drug withdrawal after birth. Researchers described a withdrawal syndrome with such characteristics as fever, breathing difficulties, convulsions, restlessness, yawning, high-pitched excessive crying, and vomiting. During withdrawl these babies are often treated with a soothing medicine, such as paregoric, to reduce pain. The severity of symptoms appears to depend on the amount of heroin taken by the mother during pregnancy. One study (Schulman, 1969) of infants born with heroin withdrawal symptoms found that after withdrawal their sleep patterns differed greatly from the normal sleep pattern of a newborn. They had greater variability in heart rates, more rapid eye movements, and no truly quiet sleep, all of which indicated possible damage to the central nervous system.

However, another study (Blinick, Wallach, and Jerez, 1969) of one hundred babies born to addicts casts doubt on the findings reported above that link heroin addiction with pregnancy complications and withdrawal symptoms in the infant. As the Blinick group points out, it is difficult to blame heroin for the maternal complications of pregnancy, since they may also result from malnutrition, infection, lack of prenatal care, and poverty. No controlled studies have been conducted that compare the occurrence of complications of pregnancy among addicted and nonaddicted women from the same social class.

The mothers of the one hundred babies in this study were probably the worst specimens of motherhood an expert in prenatal development could imagine. Many suffered from malnutrition and infections such as syphilis, and they were heavy smokers. Several of them earned their living through prostitution. Among them were some who suffered also from other threats to a favorable pregnancy, such as cancer, anemia, hepatitis, and diabetes. One mother was over forty, and another had previously given birth to ten babies.

Amazingly enough, eighty-eight of the one hundred mothers gave uncomplicated birth to healthy babies, as measured by the Apgar test which rates such factors as crying, breathing, and color at birth. The main problem was low birth weight, but this is also associated with smoking and poverty. Only two babies from a larger study of 230 babies (Blatman, cited in *Proceedings, Third Methadone Conference*, 1971) had congenital defects (defects present at birth). This rate would be considered low in a more normal, unaddicted population.

The first view discussed above was that since heroin, like alcohol and nicotine from cigarettes, passes through the placenta and reaches the unborn baby, the offspring of addicted mothers must have to undergo withdrawal after birth. The Blinick group feels, however, that "placental transfer of narcotics prior to and during labor is poorly understood and the conclusions of experimentation are open to doubt. This is primarily due to the lack of accurate biochemical tests for the determination of minute amounts of opiates in blood and fetal tissues" (p. 1001). Since the one hundred babies born to addicted mothers are known to have suffered from low birth weight and other signs of immaturity, it is possible that the symptoms that are being attributed to "heroin withdrawal" may instead be the result of an immature nervous system. The pediatrician (Blatman) who treated the 230 infants feels they should not be labeled as addicts, because there is no real proof that they are addicted. According to him, to say that babies of addicts show evidence of a "withdrawal syndrome" is an undesirable usage of the term that should be eliminated.

Thus, in summary, it appears that some babies born to addicted mothers are in very good health, while other babies suffer a handicap. It has not yet been determined what proportion of this handicap is due to the heroin and what proportion is due to such detrimental factors as malnutrition, infection, and disease.

Methadone

It has been reported that methadone, which is used as a substitute for heroin addiction, is also prenatally addicting (Javate, cited in Methadone addiction in babies, 1972). A study of twenty-three babies born to methadone-addicted mothers found that seventeen of the babies suffered from what might be called withdrawal symptoms at birth. These babies were irritable, twitched violently, and suffered from cold sweats. Hospital treatment to free them from the effects of prenatal addiction to methadone lasted as long as ninety days.

Research on the question of possible damage to the fetus when the mother is on a methadone-maintenance program has shown that "the rate of congenital malformations among babies born to mothers taking high doses of methadone both before and during pregnancy does not differ significantly from the rate to be expected among nonaddicted mothers of the same age, color, and socioeconomic status" (Brecker, 1972).

A study done at Beth Israel Medical Center in New York on nineteen babies born to mothers on methadone maintenance is typical of the general findings (Blatman, cited in *Proceedings, Third National Conference on Methadone Treatment,* 1971). Pregnancy for the mothers of these babies was uneventful, with no more birth complications than would be found in a comparable nonaddicted group. There were, however, two main deviations from normality among the babies. First, while few of the babies were born early, one-third of them had low birth weight, which is, of course, a handicap. This is about the same proportion that is found in mothers addicted to heroin, but it is not known how or to what extent heroin and methadone contribute to the problem. Second, eleven of the nineteen babies were born with hyperirritability, but Blatman suggests this is not the same condition as the withdrawal symptoms reported in the Javate work. Blatman feels this hyperirritability may be related to low birth weight or to other factors unrelated to methadone. There is obviously a current disagreement between researchers regarding the nature and cause of the "hyperirritability" observed in babies born to heroin- and methadone-addicted mothers.

Marijuana

Marijuana or "pot" is derived from cannabis, which consists of the dried parts of the hemp plant. The existing research regarding the effect of marijuana on prenatal development does not present a clear-cut picture. One problem has been to find, for experimental purposes, two groups of similar subjects where one group uses marijuana and the other does not. Thus, much research has been conducted with animals. The results indicate a relationship (among animals) between the use of marijuana during pregnancy and a reduced growth rate of the fetus as well as the incidence of physical defects such as phocomelia in the developing infant (*Marihuana-hashish epidemic and its impact on United States Security,* 1974). Testimony in this report points out that

these animal studies cannot be accurately transferred to humans because of obvious differences in the high doses employed and the mode of administration utilized. However, it is apparent that there is a potential risk in cannabis use during pregnancy, and that, at present, there are no adequate studies of women who have used cannabis during pregnancy with relation to the health of their children. [p. 119]

Other testimony in the same government report suggests that since the number of chromosomes decreases in the body cells of marijuana smokers, it also seems logical to expect problems with germ cell production, genetic mutations, and birth defects. However, little is definitely known about the effects of marijuana in these areas.

There is also some question regarding the effect of marijuana smoking on male fertility, as measured by the production of testosterone, which is the principal male sex hormone. While one study (Kolodny, Masters, Kolodner, and Toro, 1974) indicates that intensive use of marijuana results in decreased testosterone production, another study (Mendelson, Kuehnle, Ellingboe, and Babor, 1974) did not find an association between chronic marijuana use and decreased testosterone level.

In summary, the effects of marijuana on prenatal development have not yet been determined. Additional research is needed in this area before definite conclusions can be reached.

LSD

The use of LSD (lysergic acid diethylamide) now appears to have decreased, but the effect of LSD on prenatal development is still an open question. It has been stated that the use of LSD by parents results in chromosomal abnormalities in their offspring. However, one large study (Lubs and Ruddle, 1970) at Yale University indicates that LSD usage by parents is at most a trivial factor in the birth of babies with chromosomal abnormalities. In a study of 4,500 consecutive births only twenty-two babies showed visible chromosomal abnormalities, and none of the parents of these babies reported having taken LSD. Thus the researchers concluded that about 20,000 babies with visible chromosomal damage are born yearly in the United

States to parents who have not taken LSD. Interestingly enough, all fourteen babies whose parents reported taking LSD had normal chromosomes.

In reviewing the research on the effects of LSD on prenatal development, it appears necessary to draw a distinction between studies in which the mother and/or father took LSD *before* the time of conception and those studies in which LSD was taken by the mother *during* pregnancy. The latter studies almost always involve animals, because it would, of course, be unethical to deliberately administer LSD to pregnant women when the consequences for prenatal development are unknown.

In one animal study (Kato, 1970) four rhesus monkeys were given LSD during pregnancy. All four of the mothers showed temporary chromosomal damage which later repaired itself. All of the mothers had late deliveries. One of the babies showed no significant chromosome damage, but the other three offspring died immediately after birth.

Two studies with somewhat different conclusions (Berlin and Jacobson, 1970; McGlothlin, Sparkes, and Arnold, 1970) were reported in the same issue of the *Journal of the American Medical Association,* and both are concerned with babies whose parents used LSD before conception.

The Berlin and Jacobson study was concerned with the effects of LSD on 127 pregnancies among 112 women. At least one and usually both of the parents admitted taking LSD before or after conception. Out of the 127 pregnancies there were only 62 live births. Six of the infants were obviously congenitally abnormal at birth, and one died at the age of nine hours.

All of the fathers of the six abnormal infants admitted taking LSD before or around the time of conception. Five of the six mothers of the abnormal infants admitted taking

LSD within one month of conception, but only two mothers actually took LSD during the crucial first three months of pregnancy.

The other sixty-five pregnancies ended in abortion. Not all of the aborted fetuses could be studied, as many of the abortions were done illegally. However, it was found that four of the fourteen therapeutically aborted fetuses were abnormal. The percentage of abnormal fetuses in the case of the spontaneous abortions is not at all unusual, because spontaneous abortion is one of nature's ways of improving the chances of normal babies being born.

Some of the parents of the abnormal infants had taken LSD several hundred times, but other parents said they had taken only a few doses. Six of the women users of LSD were followed through subsequent pregnancies. All six of their first pregnancies had resulted in a normal infant, but eight later pregnancies ended in four abnormal fetuses.

The authors refused to conclude that their findings established LSD as a mutagen. The major reason for their hesitancy was that the women in this study were not ideal candidates for motherhood anyway. They constituted a very high-risk obstetric population for many of the reasons previously discussed in this book: 81 percent smoked, 25 percent used narcotics, 36 percent had undergone extensive X-ray investigation for abdominal complaints, and many suffered from infectious diseases and malnutrition. One of the researchers concluded, "All I can say is that birth defects are more common among these children. The rate of central nervous system defect was about 16 times that in the general population" (p. 1447).

In contrast to the Berlin and Jacobson study, the McGlothlin study found a lower incidence of birth defects. Their study of 120 live births to LSD users involved few parents who had used LSD in high dosages over a long period of time, and only 12 of the mothers in their study actually took LSD during pregnancy. One hundred and six of the 120 babies were born in good health with no obvious birth defects. Ten babies were born early, seven babies showed minor defects which "ran in the family," and four babies had minor birth defects, but these percentages are much like what would be expected among babies born to parents who never used LSD. Thus the McGlothlin group concluded that parental use of LSD did not appear to be related to birth defects in their children.

However, the spontaneous abortion rate among LSD users was higher than would be found in a population of non-LSD users—15 percent higher in mothers who took LSD medicinally and 50 percent higher among mothers who took nonmedicinal LSD (usually black-market LSD). The rate was lower when only the father had taken LSD. The McGlothlin group thus concluded that the use of LSD by mothers before conception might increase the occurrence of spontaneous abortions, although the data did not establish a clear-cut causal relationship.

While the results of the McGlothlin study are somewhat less incriminating than the Berlin and Jacobson study (possibly because a smaller percentage of the McGlothlin mothers and fathers actually took LSD around the time of conception or during pregnancy), neither of the studies reliably answers the question regarding possible detrimental effects of LSD taken by the mother during pregnancy. The advice regarding the use of drugs during pregnancy given by *Consumer Reports* (Drugs in pregnancy: are they safe?, 1967) must, therefore, apply to LSD as well as to all other drugs:

No chemical known to science has been proved to be entirely harmless for all pregnant women and their babies during all stages of pregnancy. Hence, do not take any drug during pregnancy unless there is a specific medical need for it.

If there *is* a medical need, however, and if your physician prescribes a drug to meet that need, take it scrupulously, in the amounts and at the times specified. Don't increase or lower the dose; don't discontinue sooner or continue longer than directed. Remember that your unborn baby's health can be adversely affected by your failure to take a needed drug as well as by your indulgence in unprescribed medication.

If you are pregnant or potentially pregnant, be sure to tell your doctor so whenever he is prescribing a drug for you. If your regular doctor refers you to someone else while you are pregnant or potentially pregnant, be sure to tell the second doctor, too.

During pregnancy and potential pregnancy, curtail the use of over-the-counter "home remedies" as well as drugs available only on a doctor's prescription. Even common self-prescribed medicines like aspirin, for example, should be taken sparingly—except on your doctor's advice. The same goes for vitamin preparations.

Interpret the term "drugs" broadly to include many things besides oral preparations and injections—for example, lotions and ointments containing hormones or other drugs that may be absorbed through the skin; vaginal douches, suppositories and jellies; rectal suppositories; medicated nose drops; and so on.

A number of drugs exert their adverse effects during the first weeks following a missed menstrual period—the weeks when you are likely to be wondering whether you are pregnant. Hence discontinue all self-prescribed remedies within a few days after an expected menstrual period fails to occur, and recheck with your doctor concerning drugs prescribed for you previously.

Mothers who breast-feed their babies should continue to exercise prudence until weaning time. Numerous drugs taken by the mother are secreted in her milk and reach the nursing baby. [p. 435]

Diseases

Diseases, as well as drugs, are easily transmitted from the mother to the fetus. Again, in accordance with the principle of critical periods, the timing of the disease seems to be more crucial than the degree to which the mother has the disease. A mild case of rubella can be as damaging to the fetus as a severe case. In the words of one article (Adams, Heath, Imagawa, Jones, and Shear, 1956):

It is the mild or inapparent illnesses which we believe may be responsible for damage to the fetus when the mother has those infections early in the course of her pregnancy. Although the infection may be extremely mild for the mother, it may not be so mild for the fetus which is in the early stages of morphogenesis [differentiation of the body structure] with growth taking place at an extremely rapid rate. [pp. 109–110]

It also is now known (Thong, Steele, Vincent, Hensen, and Bellanti, 1973) that, at least in the case of German measles, women's natural cell-mediated immunity (an important defense against viral infections) is lowered during pregnancy. According to the Thong group, reduced cell-mediated immunity during pregnancy may be a desirable maternal response to protect the fetus from rejection, but it also exposes the mother to a greater risk of infection. Their study found the reduced immunity to be only temporary, with full immunity returning after pregnancy. It is possible that immune defenses against all viruses are weakened during pregnancy, because pregnant women often have unusually severe cases of polio, hepatitis, and other viral infections.

German Measles (or Rubella)

German measles (or rubella) is probably the best-known example of a maternal disease that may seriously damage the fetus. For an adult the disease is usually simple and uncomplicated, but for the embryo it may have disastrous

123

consequences, since the rubella virus appears to concentrate on growing embryonic tissue.

In 1941 Dr. N. M. Gregg, an Australian opthalmologist, was the first to draw a connection between congenital cataracts and maternal German measles after examining thirteen cases of congenital cataracts in babies, all of whose mothers had suffered from German measles during pregnancy. Besides congenital cataracts other characteristics of the rubella syndrome include deafness, heart disease, microcephaly, and stunted growth. Severe mental retardation used to be considered a consequence of maternal rubella, but more recent research makes this questionable. In a study (Sheridan, 1964) of over 200 children whose mothers had rubella during the first four months of pregnancy, it was found that 30 percent of the children suffered from various abnormalities. Their intelligence, however, was apparently not affected, since the distribution of high, medium, and low intelligence scores was the same among this group as among the general population.

Rubella's threat to the developing child is strongest in the first three months of pregnancy. During the first four weeks after conception the chance of defects is about 50 percent, diminishing to 17 percent in the third month, and to almost zero after the third or fourth month (Rhodes, 1961). Miscarriage, too, may occur if rubella is contracted during the first three months of pregnancy. It is generally agreed that there is a one-out-of-three chance that a defective child will be born if the mother contracts rubella during the first four months of pregnancy, and, because the chances for a normal birth are so poor, many authorities feel justified in ending the pregnancy. If maternal rubella occurs after the fourth month and especially during the last trimester of pregnacy, the child does not appear to be harmed in any way, except for the fact that the infant shows the rash of rubella. Babies born with the rash of rubella, of course, promptly start a German measles epidemic in the neonatal nursery.

A rubella vaccine is now available, but the length of immunity established by it has not yet been determined. The vaccine, which contains live viruses, cannot be given to a pregnant woman nor to a woman any later than sixty days before conception; otherwise, the effect will be the same as if she actually had rubella. Immunization programs, therefore, must center on young children who are the most likely to expose their mothers to the disease.

The most recent rubella epidemic in the United States occurred between 1963 and 1965. It affected about 50,000 children. Approximately 20,000 of these babies suffered from serious birth defects (cataracts, hearing loss, heart malformations), and 30,000 of the babies died before birth (Rugh and Shettles, 1971). Up until 1941 rubella was considered a mild inconsequential childhood disease, but it is now quite clear how devastating maternal rubella can be for the developing baby during the first trimester of pregnancy.

Measles, Mumps, Chickenpox, and Infectious Hepatitis

Most childhood viral diseases such as measles (sometimes called the "two-week" or "old-fashioned" measles), mumps, and chickenpox occur once in childhood and provide life immunity for the person. Thus there have been few reported cases of these diseases among pregnant women, and little is known about the effect on the fetus. These viral diseases, along with infectious hepatitis, have been tentatively linked with the occurrence of birth defects even though previous research has not been clear-cut. Now a thorough study (Siegel, 1973) vindicates these viruses from causing birth defects, though it is possible that they may cause other pregnancy problems.

In Siegel's study 409 pregnant women with chickenpox, measles, mumps, or hepatitis were carefully matched with 409 pregnant women who were as much like them as possible except that they were not infected with these diseases. The women were studied for the rest of their pregnancy, and their babies were studied at birth, and at ages one, two, and five years for evidence of birth defects.

A summary of this study (Four viruses vindicated from causing birth defects, 1974) reported that there was

no apparent difference in the incidence of birth defects between babies born to virus-infected mothers and those born to noninfected mothers. Their total rates were 2.2 percent and 2.3 percent respectively. The rates in specific virus and control groups varied from 1.7 percent to 1.6 percent for mumps, measles and hepatitis and from 3 percent to 3.4 percent for chickenpox. The most common defects, mental retardation and other nervous system problems, as well as multiple cases of deafness, were fairly equally distributed between babies born to infected mothers and those born to noninfected mothers and showed no distinctive concentration by period of pregnancy at onset of disease. In three cases major malformations were associated with viral disease in the last three months of pregnancy, namely mental retardation and mumps at term, deafness and chickenpox at 35 weeks of pregnancy. There was a single case of cataracts, associated with chickenpox in the eighth week of pregnancy. But on the whole, factors other than viruses appeared to have caused these isolated cases of defects because isolated defects cropped up among the control children as well. The only two cases of cardiac defects and mongolism occurred in controls. [p. 20]

Thus Siegel concludes that there is no need for expectant mothers infected with chickenpox, mumps, measles, or hepatitis to consider a therapeutic abortion, since the evidence does not indicate an increase in defective children following these four diseases. However, Siegel does not rule out other harmful prenatal effects of thse diseases. Maternal infection is said to increase the chance of early delivery and fetal deaths. In an earlier study Siegel and Feurst (1966) found that mumps, occurring during the first three months of pregnancy, resulted in an increase in fetal deaths that was due possibly to changes in the ovaries. With measles there was an increase in short-gestation-period babies. Infection with hepatitis during the last half of pregnancy resulted in an increase in the number of babies born early and in the number of fetal deaths. The effects appeared to be minimal with chickenpox.

Influenza

At present there are no studies that link the common cold with harmful effects on the developing fetus, but in the case of influenza it is a different story. One study (Rhodes, 1961) reported a 3 percent increase in the number of malformations if the mother had influenza during pregnancy.

Researchers (Coffey and Jessop, 1959) who studied the results of an Asian flu epidemic in Dublin, Ireland, in 1957, found no increase in stillbirths or early deliveries among the babies born to mothers who had contracted influenza during their pregnancies. However, the risk of malformations increased greatly the earlier in her pregnancy the mother had contracted influenza, from a risk of only 2 percent during the last trimester to a risk of over 7 percent during the first three months of pregnancy. Coffey and Jessop concluded their research by stating,

> While this figure is not alarming compared with the risk some-times claimed for rubella, and is even far short of the more con-servative estimates for the latter infection, it deserves serious no-tice because of the frequency of epidemics of influenza, the absence of lasting immunity following an attack, and, con-sequently, the high adult attack-rate during an epidemic. It strongly suggests the advisability of affording protection by vac-cination to pregnant women when an epidemic is in progress or pending. [p. 937]

Some studies suggest that pregnant women are more likely than other people to have influenza during an epi-demic and are more apt to suffer complications (Swine flu: did Uncle Sam buy a pig in a poke? 1976). For example, there appeared to be an increase in the number of sponta-neous abortions during the 1918 flu epidemic. But more recent studies do not indicate any special dangers to mothers or their unborn children during a flu epidemic.

The government-supported immunization program against swine influenza that was put into effect before the start of the 1976–1977 flu season raised the question of whether there is any special danger for expectant mothers or their babies from the immunization itself. According to one report (Swine flu: did Uncle Sam buy a pig in a poke?, 1976) pregnant women

> are not known to suffer any unusual reactions to flu vaccines, and because the swine-flu vaccine uses a killed virus, it cannot cross the placenta to harm the fetus. But fever, one of the most common side effects of immunization, may be associated with spontaneous abortions. . . . However, there's no suggestion that the degree or amount of fever would be as high as that accom-panying the natural flu. [p. 498]

An advisory committee of the Public Health Service con-cluded that pregnant women appear to have exactly the same balance of benefits and risks regarding influenza vaccination and influenza as the general population.

Syphilis and Gonorrhea

If a syphilitic mother receives penicillin treatment before the eighteenth week of her pregnancy the baby is unlikely to be affected, since fetuses under this age do not appear to be susceptible to the transmission of syphilitic spirochetes (Thompson and Grusec, 1970). However, after eighteen weeks the fetus has as much as an 80 percent chance of contracting the disease. Even if the mother manages to avoid spontaneous abortion and stillbirth, the fetus may be born deaf, blind, deformed, or mentally retarded. About 50 percent of the infected and untreated children that survive infancy will develop symptoms of syphilis during their lifetime. Thus, the extreme importance of immediate treatment of syphilis is obvious.

Gonorrhea can produce blindness in an infant if infection of the eyes occurs while the fetus is passing through the birth canal of an infected mother. The condition is easily prevented, however, through the use of silver nitrate drops placed in a neonate's eyes. This process is a legal requirement in many states. It also appears that gonorrhea can be transmitted through the placenta to the child before birth and may result in gonococcal arthritis.

Chronic Disorders

Diabetes

Diabetes is characterized by a deficiency in the supply of insulin secreted by the pancreas, so that sugar in the diet is not broken down correctly. The result is a high level of sugar in the blood and urine. Diabetes exposes the preg-

129

nant woman to a 25 percent chance of toxemia (Corner, 1961). Diabetic mothers are likely to have abnormally large fetuses that may weigh more than nine pounds; such large babies cause difficult and complicated deliveries and result in a high rate of mortality for the babies. Diabetic mothers are also more likely to have stillborns, spontaneous abortions, and babies with malformations. These problems are the result of the mother's high blood sugar level or the action of the insulin on the developing baby, or possibly to both factors. However, with suitable medical care, exercise, and diet the prenatal danger to the child may be reduced. There is a big danger to babies carried by prediabetic mothers whose condition is unknown, since the baby can be harmed by its mother's faulty sugar metabolism. The birth of an overly large baby to any woman not known to be suffering from diabetes is grounds for a thorough investigation of the cause.

Anemia

Anemia is caused by a shortage of iron, and its presence is revealed by laboratory tests that show a reduction in the number of red blood cells. Other symptoms of anemia include fatigue, irregular menstruation, and shortness of breath. The obvious treatment is an iron supplement in the diet. Anemia is especially dangerous during pregnancy, because the fetus must draw from its mother not only its fetal requirements, but also a reserve for the first year of life, since babies normally do not receive much iron in their first year's diet. Maternal anemia may thus result in a baby that will be anemic after birth.

Sickle Cell Anemia

Sickle cell anemia is found almost exclusively in the United States among blacks. About 10 percent of American blacks carry a gene for sickle cell anemia, but only one out of about 500 blacks carries two recessive genes for sickle cell anemia and thus actually suffers from the disease. (The genetic mechanisms for the inheritance of recessive characteristics such as sickle cell anemia will be discussed in detail in Chapter 6.) In this disorder the red blood cells have an inflexible sicklelike shape rather than the pliable shape of a normal red blood cell. Sickle cell shapes are beneficial in the prevention of malaria, but they are otherwise detrimental because their inflexible shape prevents them from moving easily through the blood system and thus they clot in joints and organs. This clotting results in much pain and damage to the body. Children born to women with sickle cell anemia have high mortality rates. They may be carriers of the disorder, or they may have sickle cell anemia themselves, if they receive the recessive gene for it from both parents. At present there is no cure for the disorder.

Two groups of researchers (Kan, Golbus, and Trecartin, 1976; Alter, Friedman, Hobbins, Mahoney, Sherman, McSweeney, Schwartz, and Nathan, 1976) report that it is now possible to diagnose sickle cell anemia in living human fetuses. The technique involves a process similar to amniocentesis except that a specimen of blood is withdrawn from a fetal blood vessel rather than a sample of amniotic fluid. The blood sample is then studied to determine whether the fetus has the disease. These techniques are performed on fetuses about twenty weeks old, which is about the upper limit for a therapeutic abortion.

The prenatal diagnosis of sickle cell anemia, as well as of other diseases, raises the ethical question of what to do if a fetus is found to have the disease. There are only two choices: let the diseased infant be born or abort it. Thus, the important question is: Should fetuses diagnosed for the disease be aborted? One researcher (Golbus) feels that the problem raised by learning that their developing fetus has sickle cell anemia should be handled individually by each couple, but another researcher (Alter) feels that since the test is risky it should not be performed unless the couple has already decided on an abortion if they find that their fetus has sickle cell anemia (Sickle cell anemia detected in fetuses, 1976).

Fortunately, the drugs, diseases, and chronic disorders discussed in this chapter influence only a very small proportion of expectant mothers. However, Montagu (1962) has pointed out that small as this proportion might be "it is significantly large enough to cause us to take every practical prophylactic [preventive] step to ensure optimum health in the mother, and in this way ensure the optimum conditions of development for the fetus" (p. 321).

6 Every Child's Right to Be Born Normal

It has been stated that "if a human right exists at all it is the right to be born with normal body and mind, with the prospect of developing further to fulfillment. If this is to be denied, then life and conscience are mockery and a chance should be made for another throw of the ovarian dice" (Berrill, 1968, p. 153).

"Prematurity"

Traditionally, the term "premature baby" has been used to refer to a baby that was born early (that is, born before term, which is a gestational age of 266 days from conception) or to a baby born small (weighing less than 2,500 grams, which is about 5½ pounds). When prematurity is defined in this general way, it can be considered both the cause and the result of hazards to the child's development. It is responsible for causing physical, psychological, and intellectual problems, and it results from such factors as malnutrition, inadequate prenatal care, unfavorable socioeconomic conditions, a multiple pregnancy where the uterine walls cannot expand further, excessive smoking, oxygen starvation or anoxia, emotional disturbances, drugs, some illnesses like syphilis, and noninfectious disorders. Prematurity is more common among very young women having a succession of babies, women having their first baby after the age of forty, and women with complications of pregnancy. Prematurity is also more common among first-borns than later-borns, among male than female babies, among nonwhites than whites, and among smaller women than larger women.

Even the research on prematurity presents contradictions. For example, one study (Drillien and Ellis, 1964) reported that premature babies grow faster both physically and mentally during the first two years of life, while another study (Braine, Heimer, Wortis, and Freedman, 1966) reported that the premature infant has a slower rate of mental and motor development during the first year of life. The probable explanation for these contradictory findings is that much of the research has been on prematurity as a general category, when in fact the term needed more careful definition.

In 1961 the World Health Organization attempted to clarify this situation by dividing prematures into two classifications. A low-birth-weight infant has been defined as one weighing under 5½ pounds or 2,500 grams, despite a normal period of prenatal development. Some authorities prefer an upper limit of 2,000 grams or a little over four pounds. A short-gestation-period infant has been defined as one born after a shorter-than-usual period of development in the uterus. The infant is then judged against standards for other children whose gestation periods were similar, and if its weight on this basis is low, it is called small-for-dates. According to Tanner (1970): "Clearly the prognosis for a small child born after the normal length gestation and an equally small child born after a shortened gestation may be very different. Leaving the uterus early is not in itself necessarily deleterious, whereas growing less than normally during a full uterine stay implies pathology of fetus, placenta, or mother" (p. 92).

Short-Gestation-Period Infants

A short-gestation-period infant is one who is born early, that is, from approximately twenty-eight to thirty-four weeks after conception instead of after its full development is completed at thirty-eight weeks. Such a short-gestation-period baby looks different from a full-term baby. Because it did not have all of the last two months of uterine development in which to lay down fat layers under the skin, its skin looks red and wrinkled. Its head is extra big for its tiny body. Sometimes it is too weak to suck and swallow well, and it must be fed intravenously or by stomach tube. Since the brain is not yet sufficiently developed to control all the functions of the infant, it may breathe irregularly and be unable to control its bodily temperature, thus necessitating the use of an incubator. Often the short-gestation-period infant is extremely susceptible to infection, for it is unable to increase the white blood count that is necessary to fight infection.

In the past, large amounts of oxygen were pumped into incubators in order to keep the short-gestation-period infant alive. The result was often retrolental fibrophasia, a condition that causes damage to the cells of the retina in the eye and results in permanent blindness. Since the 1953 discovery of the damaging effects of too much oxygen, smaller amounts are now used.

Babies born before the end of the usual gestation period tend to be small, but this is, of course, often explained by the shorter period of prenatal development. The development of numerous enzymes, the maturation of the nervous system, and the appearance of conditioned reflexes all seem to be on a schedule of development independent of that for birth. It has been found that the electroencephalogram (a tracing which shows the changes in electric potential produced by the brain) of a baby born at thirty-four weeks will be just like one done six weeks after birth on a baby born after twenty-eight weeks of gestation. The developmental stages of motor behavior in a baby born early, as measured by detailed neurological examination, continue to occur just as if birth did not change the course of maturation. Apparently the normal schedule of maturation is followed just as closely in the incubator as in the mother's uterus.

If the short-gestation-period infant receives proper care, it may demonstrate an accelerated "catch-up growth period" once it weighs five pounds.[1] This catch-up growth is usually completed by three years of age, by which time many short-gestation-period babies have reached average height and weight. However, even though these short-gestation-period babies may experience the catch-up phenomenon in physical growth, they do not necessarily totally catch up in all aspects of development, such as in behavioral and intellectual development.

Low-Birth-Weight Infants

In contrast to the above-mentioned short-gestation-period babies, low-birth-weight babies have quite different problems. Babies weighing between 2,000 and 2,500

---

[1]Tanner (1970: 125–129) discusses the phenomenon of "catch-up growth." He argues that the growth curve of each child is genetically determined and self-stabilizing. Even though normal growth may be temporarily slowed down by hazards such as malnutrition and illness, it is likely that the child will catch up again later if the environment becomes normal.

grams may simply be small babies born after a normal-length gestation to genetically small mothers. These babies are likely to have only slight, if any, deficits in intellectual ability and size. From birth to about six months, these smaller babies gain more weight than larger babies. The catch-up process explains why it is possible for small women to bear small babies who become large adults.

However, some of the babies weighing under 2,500 grams and especially those weighing under 2,000 grams after a normal-length gestation are more likely to have suffered some type of developmental difficulty. These low-birth-weight infants have been divided into two groups based on whether their small size was due to *internal* growth failure resulting from such factors as congenital malformations and genetic diseases, or to *external* growth failure resulting from such factors as maternal vascular disease (which may have caused a reduced blood supply to the fetus) or from maternal malnutrition (Winick, 1976). As was discussed in detail in Chapter 3, prenatal malnutrition is especially damaging, because it can result not only in lower birth weights and increased fetal mortality, but also in permanently retarded intellectual and behavioral development.

Low-birth-weight infants have a neonatal mortality rate more than twenty times greater than that of heavier infants (Shapiro, Schlesinger, and Nesbitt, 1968). The mothers of these infants are also more likely to have a higher proportion of abnormal infants in later conceptions than the mothers of larger babies. Whatever aspect of prenatal development (for example, congenital malformations, inborn errors of metabolism, other genetic diseases, abnormalities in the maternal and fetal environment such as malnutrition) kept these babies from gaining weight prenatally seems also to inhibit their later catch-up growth. Low-birth-weight babies are likely to remain always shorter and lighter in weight for their age (Cruise, 1973).

An extensive five-year study of low-birth-weight infants was carried out by Drillien and Ellis (1964), who matched, according to social class, 1,000 low-birth-weight infants with 1,000 infants of normal weight. They found that low-birth-weight infants had lower intelligence and developmental scores in their early years. In general, the lower the birth weight, the lower the intelligence. The low-birth-weight infants grew faster than infants of normal weight, both mentally and physically, during the first two years of life. However, with the possible exception of the larger infants weighing between 4½ and 5½ pounds, they still had not by age five reached the level of heavier children growing up under similar environmental circumstances, and they probably never will catch up. Drillien and Ellis also found the occurrence of severe physical abnormalities to be higher among low-birth-weight children. When maternal care was unsatisfactory, the chances of developmental problems during the preschool years increased.

The results of a University of Minnesota study (cited in Performance in school linked to birth weight, 1974) are in agreement with the Drillien and Ellis findings and indicate that children who weigh less than five pounds at birth tend to fall behind heavier children in both physical and mental development. At ages five and seven these low-birth-weight children performed less well than heavier children on traditional tests of language development, reading, spelling, mathematical skills, and intelligence. The low-birth-weight children were also far likelier to be retained in the same grade.

A common problem shared by both short-gestation-period and low-birth-weight infants is the different treatment they receive compared to that given to a more normal infant. While still in the hospital after birth, the child must often spend long periods in the unstimulating environment of an incubator, where it is separated from its parents during what is considered a critical period for the development of child and parent ties. Once the child is brought home from the hospital, the parents may isolate or overprotect the child. For fear of harming the baby they consider fragile, they may not touch and stimulate the child sufficiently. One interesting experiment (Solkoff, Yaffe, Weintraub, and Blase, 1969) provided five minutes of daily tactile stimulation (stroking of the body by the nurses) for ten days for this kind of infant, while a control group of similar infants was left alone. It was found that the stroked infants were healthier and gained more weight than the control infants.

In summary, the general term "prematurity," as defined by both short gestation period (born less than thirty-four weeks after conception) and low birth weight (weighing under 5½ pounds after a normal period of gestation)—and after controlling for such factors as social class, maternal characteristics, and race—has been associated with a long list of disadvantages. Intellectual deficiencies, perceptual-motor disabilities, brain injury, immature speech, cerebral palsy, visual defects, and difficulty with abstract reasoning are some of the disadvantages.[2] It seems obvious that the best way to increase a child's chances of being born normal is to reduce the incidence of both short-gestation-period and low-birth-weight babies by eliminating as many as

[2]Fitzgerald and McKinney (1970) provide references for this list of problems associated with short-gestation-length and low-birth-weight babies.

possible of the causes, such as excessive smoking, malnutrition, and inadequate prenatal medical care.

"Postmaturity" and Oversized Babies

A "postmature infant" has been defined (Montagu, 1962) as one born two weeks or more beyond the expected date. Approximately 12 percent of births occur two weeks after the due date, and 4 percent are born three weeks or more late. An oxytocin test makes it possible to determine whether it is safe for a particular baby to undergo the stress of labor, but it does not necessarily tell that a pregnancy is overdue.[3] Because the placenta sometimes stops functioning after the due date and the baby is forced to provide its own nourishment, a postmature infant is often smaller in weight than a full-term baby. Postmature infants, for whom cerebral hemorrhage and asphyxia (suffocation) are frequent causes of death, have a mortality rate three times that for normal term babies.

The previous section makes it clear that low-birth-weight babies are more likely to be mentally slow than average-weight babies. A study (Babson, Henderson, and Clark, 1969) of oversized infants (males weighing over 9 lb. 6 oz., and females weighing over 9 lbs. at birth) found that at age four these babies also were more likely to be mentally slow than a control group of four-year-olds who were of normal weight at birth. Both the control and experimental group children came from socioeconomic-level homes where the mothers averaged about eleven years of schooling. The children were tested with the Stanford-Binet intelligence test at age four. The researchers concluded that further investigation is necessary of fetal, maternal, and environmental factors that might have caused these results.

[3]Montagu (1964: 166–167) describes the oxytocin test.

The Prevention of Birth Defects

Approximately 94 percent of the live births in the United States result in a normal, healthy baby. The remaining 6 percent are born defective, and for a variety of reasons many conceptions end in death before birth. Consider the following facts:[4]

1. Out of the approximately 3.3 million babies born yearly in the United States, 700 each day, or one every two minutes, are marred by a defect such as cleft palate, Mongolism, split spine, or other birth defects.

2. As many as fifteen million living Americans suffer from some birth defect. Three million of these people are mentally retarded.

3. An estimated 500,000 embryos are conceived each year, but fail to make it to birth.

4. There are almost 1½ million preschool children in the United States who were born with defects, who spend a total of six million days yearly in the hospital, and whose medical care costs at least $180 million annually.

5. Approximately 10 percent of the families in this country have had direct experience with a defective child.

6. An estimated 18,000 infants die each year before their first birthday due to birth defects.

7. An estimated 20 million future life years will be lost, this year alone, due to genetic defects.

8. Approximately one-fifth of all birth defects result from defects in particular chromosomes or genes.

9. At least 50 percent of all mentally defective children are the result of exposure to an abnormal prenatal environment.

10. At least half of the defective babies result from inad-

[4]The source for statements 1–7, 9, 10 is Rugh and Shettles (1971: 139–145).

equate prenatal care during pregnancy, and, more importantly, the cause of their defects could have been prevented.

There are two kinds of birth defects. A hereditary defect is one that is inherited in the genes or the chromosomes from the parents and can be passed on to future children. A child may be born an albino (an albino has a deficiency of coloring matter resulting in abnormally white skin and hair and pink eyes), because it inherited two recessive genes for albinism from its parents. The second kind of defect results from an event occurring after conception and the defect is present at birth: a child may be born with flipper arms, for example, because its mother took thalidomide tablets during pregnancy. This kind of defect cannot be passed on to the next generation, because it is not carried in the genes or chromosomes. A defect like blindness, however, may be a hereditary defect due to inheriting genes for blindness from the parents, or it may be a defect resulting from the mother contracting German measles during her pregnancy. Both of these defects would be congenital defects, since they would be present in the child at birth.

Fetology is a whole new area of medical science which is concerned with techniques for diagnosing and treating fetal illnesses and defects. Teratology is the special area of this science for the study of birth defects. More than 1,700 kinds of abnormalities that are caused by mistakes in body formation or functioning have already been identified. These faults result from heredity, or are induced by drugs, viruses, or exposure to X-rays. They range from extra fingers or toes to major defects like deafness, blindness, mental retardation, and physical paralysis. Some defects cause early death, and other result in lifelong disability. The resulting medical, economic, social, and emotional burden on both the family and society is tremendous. For example, approximately 4,000 Mongoloid children are born yearly in the United States (Friedmann, 1971). Mongoloids (children showing Down's syndrome) are a great burden to many parents and are frequently institutionalized at state expense. Often cheerful and friendly, they are also severely retarded and have a maximum intellectual age of about seven and an average life expectancy of only ten years. During that ten-year period the cost of institutional care for each one is approximately $250,000.

Most of the defects found in the approximately 250,000 abnormal babies born annually in the United States fall into one or more of the following seventeen categories (Rugh and Shettles, 1971, pp. 142–145): birthmarks, cleft palate, clubfoot, congenital heart disease (many times caused by German measles contracted by the mother in the early stages of pregnancy), cystic fibrosis, erythroblastosis (caused by the Rh factor), extra or fused fingers or toes, galactosemia (the absence of an enzyme needed to process milk sugar), genitourinary defects (possibly caused by a potassium deficiency brought on by the taking of diuretics), hydrocephaly ("water on the brain" possibly caused by prenatal infection), imperforate anus (a rectum lacking the usual opening), Mongolism (found in one out of 600 births and more common in infants born to older women perhaps because their ova have "gone stale"), phenylketonuria (known as PKU, an inherited chemical imbalance), pyloric stenosis (a blockage of the opening from the stomach into the small intestine found more frequently in males), sickle cell anemia, and split spine or spina bifida. Both hereditary influences and events occurring during the course of pregnancy are responsible for the above-mentioned kinds of birth defects.

The Genetic Basis for Birth Defects

Life begins at conception when the 23 chromosomes contained in the mother's egg merge with the 23 chromosomes contained in the father's sperm. Each new individual thus receives a total complement of 46 chromosomes. These chromosomes are further subdivided into smaller units called genes which are the carriers of the child's heredity.

It is important to note here that there are two different kinds of cells in the human body—the *body* cells and the *germ* cells from which the sperm and ova are derived. Body cells are produced by a process called mitosis in which each of the 46 chromosomes in the original cell separates in half lengthwise down the center. Each body cell thus contains 23 pairs of chromosomes and is a direct copy of the original 23 pairs of chromosomes each individual obtained from its parents.

In contrast, germ cells are produced by a process called meiosis in which certain cells in the ovaries of the mother and the testes of the father divide twice in order to produce ova and sperm with only one-half the normal number of chromosomes. Each chromosome is a double strand that occurs in the parent cell in pairs. During the first division each chromosome pair splits up, and then during the second division each chromosome splits into two parts. Each part regenerates its missing part in the next step. The result is four cells, each having a set of 23 *single* chromosomes. At conception a sperm containing 23 chromosomes unites with an egg containing 23 chromosomes, and the result is a new individual with 46 chromosomes or 23 pairs.[5]

[5]Mussen, Conger, and Kagan (1974: 75–85) provide an excellent description, stripped of genetic complexities, of hereditary transmission, or see McClearn (1970: 39–76) for a more technical discussion of these genetic processes.

This brief discussion of the mechanics of genetic transmission provides the necessary background for a discussion of the three methods of genetic transmission of birth defects—dominant and recessive genes, sex-linked defects, and chromosomal abnormalities.

Dominant and Recessive Genes

The presence or absence of some birth defects is dependent on whether the individual has dominant or recessive genes for that defect. If the individual has a *dominant* gene for a trait, that trait will appear in the individual (1) when it is paired with a similar gene, and also (2) when that gene is paired with a different gene for the trait. In the case of a *recessive* gene for a trait, that trait appears only when it is paired with a similar recessive gene. Thus an individual can be homozygous for a characteristic, meaning it inherited matching genes for this characteristic from its parents, or an individual can be heterozygous, meaning that its cells have different genes for the same trait. The presence or absence of a birth defect in these heterozygous individuals depends on whether the gene for the defect under consideration is dominant or recessive.

Phenylketonuria (PKU), which is caused by an inherited inability to metabolize phenylalanine (a component of many foods), occurs in about one in 10,000 live births. PKU provides a good example of the genetic transmission of a characteristic that depends on a single pair of genes. If left untreated, the concentration of phenylalanine in PKU victims damages the nervous system and can result in moderate to severe retardation, together with such other characteristics as temper tantrums, a stiff walk, a small head in proportion to body size, and agitated and restless behavior. It is not now possible to determine the presence of PKU by prenatal examination through amniocentesis, but

The Child before Birth

many states require the testing of newborn children for PKU. Once PKU is diagnosed, it is then possible to control its effects by feeding afflicted children a diet very low in phenylalanine.

In order to understand the transmission of PKU, let N symbolize the gene corresponding to normal metabolic ability and let p represent the gene for PKU. (Note that capital letters are used to represent dominant genes, while lower-case letters are used to represent recessive genes.) N and p thus represent the alleles, which are the different forms that this gene can take at a particular location on a chromosome. In the diagram below, which illustrates these alleles in one pair of chromosomes, the cells of both the father and mother have a gene for both N and p. Thus, when the germ cells for both parents divide, half of the father's sperm cells and half of the mother's egg cells will contain a gene for normal metabolism of phenylalanine (N), and half will contain a gene for PKU (p). As shown, each conception has four possible outcomes: NN, Np, Np, pp. Since in the case of PKU the normal gene N is dominant over the recessive gene p, the only individual who would suffer from PKU as a result of these four conception possibilities would be the one with pp genes. If the genetic selection process were perfectly random (which it is not in real life), one-half of the babies of these parents would have a genetic inheritance of Np, one-fourth of NN, and one-fourth of pp. Thus, theoretically, only one out of four of the babies of these parents would suffer from PKU.

$$Np \times Np$$
$$\downarrow$$
$$NN\ Np\ Np\ pp$$

It is also possible for the single gene producing a birth

146

defect to be dominant (rather than recessive as in the case of PKU). An example of such a dominant effect is provided by Huntington's chorea. This defect is characterized by the beginning of nervous-system degeneration in adulthood, and is accompanied by the development of unstable mental behavior. For illustration purposes let H stand for the dominant Huntington's chorea gene and n stand for the normal recessive gene. In the diagram below, which represents these alleles in one pair of chromosomes, one parent is heterozygous for Huntington's chorea (Hn), which means that this parent suffers from the disease (since the disease is genetically dominant), and one parent is homozygous for the disease (nn). Thus there are four conception possibilities: Hn, Hn, nn, nn. In this situation, if the genetic selection process were perfectly random, one-half of the babies would have the genetic inheritance for Huntington's chorea (Hn) and one-half would not (nn). In other words, if the disease is a dominant one, such as Huntington's chorea and one parent carries one gene for the disease, the risk of disease to the fetus is 50 percent. Huntington's chorea cannot yet be detected prenatally through the process of amniocentesis, because biochemical tests for this disease and other dominant diseases are not available. Tissue-culture examination in the laboratory of the cells in the amniotic fluid reveal only chromosomal abnormalities, such as those found in Down's syndrome, but Huntington's chorea is caused by one of the hundreds of thousands of genes found on a single chromosome.

$$Hn \times nn$$
$$\downarrow$$
$$Hn \; Hn \; nn \; nn$$

Sex-linked Defects

One of the twenty-three pairs of chromosomes found in every normal person determines the person's sex. The determination of sex occurs by chance in the following way (McClearn, 1970). The female sex chromosomes are always XX. This means that the XX chromosomal pair are equal in terms of microscopic appearance and in terms of having the same genes arranged in the same order. In any division of the female germ cell prior to mating with the male sperm, the female part or egg will always be X. However, the male sex chromosomes are paired XY. Through a microscope the inequality of the members of this chromosome pair can be seen. The longer of the sex chromosomes is called the X chromosome and the shorter one is the Y chromosome. The smaller Y chromosome appears to contain none (or but a few) of the genes found on the X chromosome. Thus a recessive gene on the X chromosome of a male cannot have its effects masked by the presence of a dominant gene on the Y chromosome. When the division of the male germ cell occurs, the resulting sperm may be X or it may be Y. When the female egg merges with an X-bearing sperm, the nuclei of the egg and sperm will fuse XX, and the offspring will be female. When the female egg is penetrated by a Y-bearing sperm, the offspring will be XY or male.

Some genetic diseases are sex-linked. This means they are caused by mutations on the X chromosomes and therefore more commonly affect males. The bleeding disease hemophilia is the best known of the sex-linked diseases. Hemophilia is caused by a deficiency in one of the protein factors required for normal clotting of the blood. The result is prolonged and often uncontrollable bleeding at the site of any bruise or injury to the body.

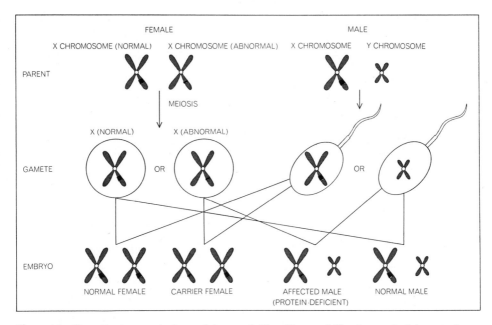

FEMALE

X CHROMOSOME (NORMAL)   X CHROMOSOME (ABNORMAL)

MALE

X CHROMOSOME   Y CHROMOSOME

PARENT

MEIOSIS

X (NORMAL)   X (ABNORMAL)

GAMETE   OR   OR

EMBRYO

NORMAL FEMALE   CARRIER FEMALE   AFFECTED MALE   NORMAL MALE
(PROTEIN-DEFICIENT)

Figure 6. Genetic transmission of hemophilia. Hemophilia is carried by mothers who have a defective gene for a blood-clotting protein in one of their X chromosomes. Daughters (XX) of these mothers have a 50 percent chance of being a carrier (but they almost never have the disease because they have at least one normal X chromosome). However, any sons (XY) of a carrier will have a 50 percent chance of having the disease, since they lack the normal gene on the second X chromosome which would mask the effect of the gene for hemophilia. From ''Prenatal Diagnosis of Genetic Disease'' by T. Friedmann, *Scientific American,* November, 1971, 225: 34–42. Copyright © 1971 by Scientific American, Inc. All rights reserved.

The genetic transmission of hemophilia has been explained by Friedmann (1971) in this way (see also Figure 6):

An ovum from a female carrier of hemophilia will have either a normal X chrososome or a defective one. After fertilization half of all the resulting males will receive as their only X chromosome the one carrying the mutant gene. Since there is no normal copy of the gene from the father such males will express the defect fully. (The father must pass his Y chromosome in order for the fetus to be male.) The other males will be normal, since they have by chance received the normal X chromosome from the mother. [p. 34]

149

Prenatal determination of the sex of the child can rule out some possibilities for the presence of hemophilia. A smear, made of the fetal cells collected from the amniotic fluid during amniocentesis, shows the presence or absence of the sex chromatin body, which is a condensation of nuclear material possessed only by female cells. The presence of a female fetus in utero almost totally rules out the possibility of hemophilia, although it is possible for the female to carry the disease without being afflicted with it, and, in exceedingly rare cases, it is possible for a female to be a hemophiliac—if the father suffers from hemophilia and the mother is a carrier for the disease. A male fetus, however, may be either afflicted or normal. In order to prevent the birth of males afflicted with hemophilia, it would be necessary to screen all possibly hemophilic pregnancies and to abort all male fetuses since there is no way at present to distinguish in utero the male fetuses afflicted with the disease from those who are normal.

Chromosomal Abnormalities

During the process of meiosis, in which the germ cells split, separate, and reproduce themselves, things can go wrong. A pair of chromosomes may fail to separate, so that one of the new germ cells has one extra chromosome and the other has a missing one. Sometimes these abnormalities involve the sex chromosomes. For example, individuals with only a single Y sex chromosome have not been found, but if the missing chromosome is the Y sex chromosome in the father's sperm cell, then the single X condition (symbolized XO) results in a child with Turner's syndrome. These children are ostensibly female, but as adults they will lack secondary sex characteristics, such as breast development; they tend to be short and to have mild-to-moderate mental retardation.

There are other kinds of sex chromosomal abnormalities as well, such as those involving the presence of three sex chromosomes.[6] The XYY "supermale" provides an example of one kind of combination. The XYY males tend to be unusually tall, and may show aggressive and violent behavior, as suggested by some early research. A more recent large-scale study (Witkin, Sarnoff, Schulsinger, Bakkestrom, Christiansen, Goodenough, Hirshhorn, Lundsteen, Owen, Philip, Rubin, and Stocking, 1976) suggests that males with the XYY abnormality are characterized by lower intelligence scores and educational levels as well as by a higher rate of conviction for crimes than normal XY males—but the crimes were generally not acts of aggression. The researchers caution that their findings do not mean that intelligence is controlled by the Y chromosome, but rather that an extra Y somehow causes a developmental lag that can result in lowered intelligence. The Witkin group emphasizes that no evidence was found linking an extra Y chromosome to aggression.

Another kind of sex chromosomal trisomy involves males with XXY chromosomes. The Witkin group found the characteristics of these men similar to those of the XYY men. Their crime rate was higher than the XY men studied, but lower than that of the XYY men. Again, the men with this sex chromosome complement were not found to be especially aggressive. The similarities betwen the XYY men and the XXY men suggest that, at least for the characteristics studied, the consequences of an extra Y chromosome may not be specific to that chromosomal abnormality, but may also result from an extra X chromosome.

Individuals with an XXX chromosomal pattern have also been described. However, a clear clinical picture of

[6]McClearn (1970) offers an interesting discussion of the many types of sex chromosomal abnormalities and their resulting characteristics.

their characteristics has not yet emerged (McClearn, 1970).

Among chromosomal abnormalities that do not involve the sex chromosomes, the most common is Down's syndrome or Mongolism. These children are born with large folds of skin above the eye that give the child an Oriental appearance—thus the term Mongolism. Other characteristics include a low level of intelligence, a short and stocky appearance, and a life span, frequently, of no more than ten or twelve years.

Downs's syndrome is caused by a defect in the separation of chromosomes during the process of meiosis in the developing egg. This defect results in the formation of an egg with two No. 21 chromosomes (each of the 23 pairs of chromosomes has been numbered by researchers) rather than the usual single No. 21 chromosome (see Figure 7). When this egg is fertilized by a normal sperm (which has a single No. 21 chromosome), the result is an offspring with three No. 21 chromosomes and a total of 47 instead of the normal 46 chromosomes. Figure 8 shows the chromosomal analysis obtained through amniocentesis for a developing female fetus suffering from Down's syndrome. This type of chromosomal abnormality accounts for more than 95 percent of all children born with Down's syndrome.[7]

For some as yet unexplained reason, failure of the No. 21 chromosome to separate during meiosis is more apt to occur among older women. A forty-year-old pregnant woman is ten times more likely to have an affected baby than is a twenty-five-year-old woman. It has been stated (Friedmann, 1971) that

one of the clearest current indications for amniocentesis is advanced maternal age, since that is associated with the greatly

[7]McClearn (1970) gives the genetic explanation for the other 5% of the cases with Down's syndrome.

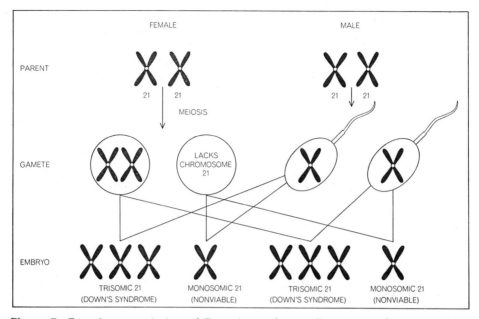

Figure 7. Genetic transmission of Down's syndrome. Down's syndrome or Mongolism results when the chromosomes do not separate normally during the process of meiosis; as a result, some ova do not have any No. 21 chromosomes and some ova have two No. 21 chromosomes. The ovum lacking the No. 21 chromosome will not survive, even when fertilized by a normal sperm. When the ovum with the extra No. 21 chromosome is fertilized by a normal sperm, the result is a fertilized ovum with a total of 47 chromosomes that will develop abnormally. From "Prenatal Diagnosis of Genetic Disease" by T. Friedmann, *Scientific American,* November, 1971, 225:34–42. Copyright © 1971 by Scientific American, Inc. All rights reserved.

increased risk of Down's syndrome. It has been estimated that if all pregnancies in women 35 years or age or older were evaluated by *in utero* detection methods, the rate of occurrence of this disease would be reduced to half the present level if selective abortion were practiced. Such age criteria, however, do not apply in many genetic disorders. [p. 38]

Dominant and recessive genes, sex-linked defects, and chromosomal abnormalities are thus the three most common mechanisms responsible for genetic defects. The new techniques of genetic counseling and amniocentesis make it possible to reduce or eliminate the occurrence of genetic

153

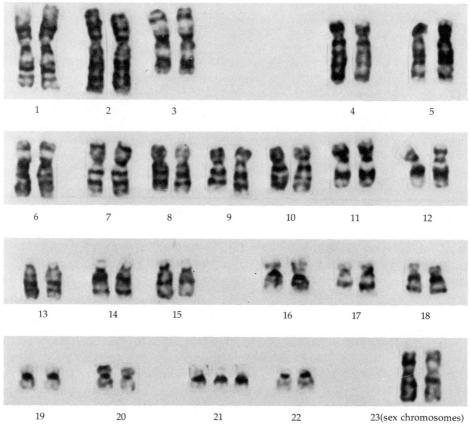

Figure 8. Chromosomal analysis of cells of child with Down's syndrome. By chromosomal analysis of cells obtained through amniocentesis it is possible to determine whether the developing child has Down's syndrome (Mongolism). This karyotype prepared by Dr. Oliver W. Jones shows an extra No. 21 chromosome, which indicates that the child will suffer from Mongolism. Note also that this child is a female, a fact made evident by the No. 23 pair of XX sex chromosomes. Courtesy of Dr. Oliver W. Jones.

defects that impose financial and emotional burdens on parents, often impose financial burdens on society, and cause suffering and death for the afflicted children. Genetic mutations, however, or "accidents," are still capable of spoiling the best laid plans of both genetic counselors and expectant parents.

Genetic Counseling and Amniocentesis

Until recently researchers and doctors could give concerned potential and expectant parents only general information about their chances of having a defective child. In the case of certain genetic defects like Mongolism, which in 95 percent of the cases results from the presence of 47 rather than 46 chromosomes, they might have been able to tell older parents, for instance, that they had one chance out of three of producing a Mongoloid child. This put the parents roughly in the position of playing Russian roulette, never knowing in which pregnancy misfortune could strike. Many parents preferred not to play the game with these odds. Now, when hereditary defects are present in a family, a new series of techniques in the field of genetic counseling makes it possible not only to predict the risks before the time of conception, but also to inform the parents whether or not a specific fetus being carried by the mother is defective. Researchers also are beginning to map the location of genes on the human chromosomes, as has already been done for the mouse, so that it will be possible to determine prenatally the presence of particular genetic defects, such as those that cause Huntington's chorea. It has even been suggested that in the future it might be possible in the prenatal child to replace defective genes with artificial substitutes.

Twenty years ago there were only a dozen birth-defect counseling centers; now there are over 150.[8] Genetic counseling is usually a three-step process that is most com-

[8]For additional information on the techniques discussed in the following section write the Medical Department, The National Foundation, 800 Second Avenue, New York, New York 10017, or write the National Genetics Foundation, 250 West 51st Street, New York, New York 10017.

monly sought by women over thirty who are concerned about their increased chances of having a defective child, by couples already having a defective child, or by couples whose family history reveals the presence of an abnormality believed to be hereditary.

To illustrate the three steps of genetic counseling an example of a twenty-two-year-old woman will be used.[9] This woman's first child was a male afflicted with Mongolism who died four days after his birth. The woman and her husband were understandably reluctant to have another child, even though their physician assured them that the tragedy was not likely to repeat itself.

After three years of indecision the parents went to a medical center specializing in genetic counseling. The genetic counselor explained to them that the chances of a 25-year-old woman having a Mongoloid child were approximately one out of 2,500, and that unless there was a genetic basis for the problem the situation was not likely to repeat itself. However, the woman was still extremely reluctant to have another child, as she kept feeling something was just not right. She requested further help.

The first step was to draw up "pedigrees," in much the same way as for purebred dogs, for both of the couple's families, going back as many generations as possible and tracing the marriages and children produced. The diagnosis for both of them was normal.

The second step was to make a chromosomal analysis of the cells of both parents. As previously discussed, chromosomes are the tiny rodlike structures in every person's body that determine how the body will develop; and a gene is a unit of a chromosome that gives one particular

[9]Described by Brody (1969) and based on a true case, this example shows the use of genetic counseling and amniocentesis.

order in the construction of a human being. It has been estimated that every normal human being carries from three to eight potentially harmful recessive genes that would result in a defective child if two such harmful genes happened to occur together (that is, if both parents carried the same recessive genes). The chances of this occurring are very small, however, except where intermarriage has been common between people of the same geographical area, race, or religion.

Some defects such as sickle cell anemia and Tay-Sachs disease are found almost exclusively among black and Jewish people, respectively, precisely because of intermarriage within each of these groups. Sickle cell anemia was discussed in Chapter 5. Tay-Sachs disease is a hereditary enzyme deficiency that occurs almost exclusively in Jewish families of eastern European descent. Approximately one out of thirty Jews of this heritage carries the Tay-Sachs gene. If two carriers should marry, there is a 25 percent chance that their child will inherit the recessive Tay-Sachs gene. Infants with this disease lack the enzyme necessary to break down fatty materials (lipids) properly. The result is a massive accumulation of lipids in nerve cells throughout the body. Afflicted infants become blind, deaf, and mentally retarded, and early death follows at age two or three. Tay-Sachs disease can be detected through amniocentesis (since the enzyme deficiency is detectable in fetal amniotic cells) or by detection of the carrier state in the parents' blood. One possible way to prevent these kinds of genetic birth defects is to encourage intermarriage of people across wide geographical, racial, and religious lines. This would decrease the chances of the same potentially harmful recessive genes being present in both marriage partners.

At the present time chromosomal analysis of cells is too expensive a procedure to be done on any widespread basis. However, it has been predicted that in the future chromosomal analysis of tissue-culture cells can be performed by computers, and everyone can carry the analysis on a card similar to a driver's license. Specific holes would be punched out on each person's card representing the genetic defects he or she carries.

In the case of the twenty-two-year-old woman and her husband discussed above, a chromosomal analysis revealed that the husband's cells were perfectly normal: he had 23 pairs of chromosomes in every cell, including the XY pair that determined his maleness. The wife, however, had only 22 *normal* pairs of chromosomes, including the XX pair marking her as a female. She had also an odd-looking twenty-third pair of chromosomes that looked under the microscope as if they had been crunched together. This marked the mother as a carrier of a rare form of Mongolism that is caused by an inherited genetic defect rather than by the much more usual genetic accident. The counselor informed the couple that in each future pregnancy they would have a one-out-of-three chance of producing a Mongoloid child.

When the couple, faced with these odds, said they did not wish to gamble on having more children, the counselor told them of the relatively new technique, amniocentesis, which makes it possible to determine early in pregnancy whether the developing child will be defective. In amniocentesis, which is performed without anesthetics and takes less than a minute, a needle thinner than the one used to draw blood samples is inserted through the maternal abdominal and uterine walls into the amniotic sac to withdraw a small amount of the fluid surrounding the un-

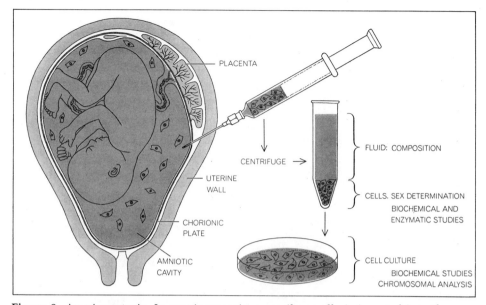

PLACENTA

CENTRIFUGE →

FLUID: COMPOSITION

UTERINE WALL

CELLS. SEX DETERMINATION
BIOCHEMICAL AND
ENZYMATIC STUDIES

CHORIONIC PLATE

AMNIOTIC CAVITY

CELL CULTURE
BIOCHEMICAL STUDIES
CHROMOSOMAL ANALYSIS

Figure 9. Amniocentesis. In amniocentesis, a sterile needle is inserted into the amniotic sac to withdraw a small amount of the amniotic fluid, which is then spun in a centrifuge to separate the fluid and cells. The amniotic-fluid cells are used in a variety of tests. From "Prenatal Diagnosis of Genetic Disease" by T. Friedmann, *Scientific American,* November, 1971, 225:34–42. Copyright © 1971 by Scientific American, Inc. All rights reserved.

born child (see Figure 9). Ultrasonic scanning is used to locate the fetus and placenta to avoid puncturing it. Because the amniotic fluid, which is made up in part from fetal urine and respiratory secretions, also has suspended in it cells shed from the fetal skin, mouth, respiratory system, kidneys, and bladder in the course of swallowing and excreting, it has been said (Friedmann, 1971) that it provides something like a road map to the kind of child developing in the uterus.

After the sample of amniotic fluid has been withdrawn it is spun in a centrifuge to separate substances of different densities. The liquid part of the sample is studied for biochemical abnormalities which are present in the urine and other excretions of the fetus.[10] The remaining cells are grown on a nutritive media for a period of two to six weeks and are then examined microscopically to determine any possible genetic abnormality of the chromosome pattern. The sixteenth week of gestation is the optimum time for amniocentesis, since by that time enough amniotic fluid has accumulated to provide a useful sample, the fetus is still small enough that it is unlikely to be damaged, and sufficient time remains to grow and analyze the cell culture and, if found necessary, to perform a therapeutic abortion.

Amniocentesis has been used since the early 1960s in Scandinavia to determine whether a developing child is chromosomally abnormal. If abnormality was found, liberal abortion laws permitted therapeutic abortion. Because of the more restrictive abortion laws found until recently in the United States, amniocentesis was mainly used to measure the amount of red-blood-cell breakdown products in the amniotic fluid so that the danger of Rh incompatibility to a developing fetus could be monitored.

At present genetic diseases that are due to extra, broken, or missing chromosomes can be detected through amniocentesis. Second, it is also possible to detect certain diseases resulting from inborn errors of body chemistry (biochemical abnormalities) in the body excretions that appear in the amniotic fluid. According to one authority (Laurence, 1974), "To date, about 60 inherited metabolic diseases are known where the actual defect has been identified and has been shown to be present in the amniotic-fluid cells, or where some identifiable product is present in

[10]See, for example, Brady (1973: 88–98), for an interesting discussion of the research leading to "new tests for detecting adult carriers and for prenatal genetic diagnosis that make it possible to control the incidence of 10 usually fatal lipid-storage diseases caused by inherited enzyme deficiencies," such as Tay-Sachs disease and Gaucher's disease.

the cells or amniotic fluid" (p. 940). However, even with amniocentesis it has not been possible to detect developmental abnormalities which result from events occurring after conception (such as congenital heart disease), since such defects are not present in the chromosomes.

Now with an instrument called the fetoscope (or endoscope) physicians can look directly at the unborn child to check for defects that would not show up in cell analysis (Hobbins and Mahoney, 1974; Chang, Hobbins, Cividalli, Frigoletto, Mahoney, Kan, and Nathan, 1974). To use the fetoscope the uterine wall is punctured as in amniocentesis, but, with this technique, on the end of the needle is a fiberoptic instrument through which the physician can look at the fetus. The instrument also has a side arm hold through which another needle can be brought down for taking a fetal blood sample. Since it is not possible to determine the presence of sickle cell anemia, for instance, through regular amniocentesis, the prenatal diagnosis of this disease (as discussed in Chapter 5) is accomplished by analysis of a blood sample acquired through the use of the side arm hold on a fetsocope. If the fetoscope had been available in the early 1960s during the thalidomide scare, it would have been possible to determine, by actually looking at the fetus, whether the developing baby was deformed.

A third area of information to be gained from amniocentesis is determination of the sex of the child. As discussed earlier in this chapter, a smear of the fetal cells from the amniotic fluid shows the presence or absence of the sex chromatin body which is found only in females. Thus in the case of a sex-linked defect like hemophilia (which generally only males have but females carry), it might be decided to abort the male children of a woman who is a genetic carrier of this disease. However, since the female children of a woman who is a carrier for hemophilia have a 50 percent chance of themselves being carriers, it might be better for such a woman and her mate to adopt children.

Some physicians are reluctant to use amniocentesis. The National Institute of Child Health is now conducting an extensive study, through a newly organized Amniocentesis Registry, to compare the long-term effects among 1,040 women who underwent amniocentesis with the outcome of 992 pregnancies among women who did not have the procedure (Brody, 1977). Preliminary results indicate amniocentesis did not result in increases in miscarriages, stillbirths, short-gestation-period babies, fetal injuries, or in birth defects (other than those detected by the procedure). At birth the babies in both groups were equally healthy and by age one there was no difference in development. Overall, amniocentesis was found to be more than 99 percent accurate in predicting the presence of a defective child.

Data from several smaller, earlier studies indicated certain risks for amniocentesis (Etzioni, 1973). Between 1 and 2 percent of the women undergoing amniocentesis will have a spontaneous abortion later—but some abortions might have occurred anyway. About 3 percent of the women will suffer an infection—which in most cases responds to antibiotics. In 8 to 10 percent of the cases bleeding may occur—but it is usually not serious. There is no record of maternal fatality, and in only two recorded cases was the fetus itself punctured. There is no evidence at present to support the claim that a child's intelligence or health may be affected by amniocentesis. Researchers in the field agree that any couple with problems for which amniocentesis might provide an answer should be told of the risks entailed by amniocentesis and of the risks it allows them to avoid, and that the decision for or against amniocentesis should be left to the parents rather than made for them by the physician.

Now, to return to the case of the couple described above and to the third step of their genetic counseling. After learning about the possibilities in amniocentesis they had decided to have another child, and returned to the genetic counselor's office for further examination when the wife was in her sixteenth week of pregnancy. After amniocentesis, four weeks were required for an anlysis of the cells in the fluid. The couple reported that it was the longest month of their lives before the counselor called back to report that they could expect the arrival of a healthy baby. This prediction was proved correct with the birth of a healthy and normal daughter. The couple is now eager for a second child and has requested the application of amniocentesis to all future pregnancies.

With the increasing use of amniocentesis, it has been pointed out (Friedmann, 1971) that

intriguing developments in our legal concepts of the unborn child seem imminent, since there are certain to be legal tests of the liability of parents and others for offspring born with genetically determined handicaps that are predictable. Such "wrongful life" suits have already been brought on behalf of illegitimate infants and some infants born with severe developmental defects due to prenatal infection with syphilis and German measles. Similar suits involving genetic diseases will soon test the concept that we—as parents, physicians and human beings—have obligations to the unborn to protect them from the likelihood of genetically determined defects. One may hope that advances in other social institutions will at the same time help us to resolve our individual and societal attitudes toward life, born and unborn. [p. 42]

Sex Determination

Not all expectant parents want to know the sex of their child before its birth. Some still prefer to be surprised. In the fortunate cases where amniocentesis reveals a healthy child is developing, many physicians prefer to tell the parents only that they can expect a healthy child rather than reveal the sex of the child. Otherwise it is a little like opening a Christmas present before the twenty-fifth of December. But in families with a history of sex-linked defects, such as hemophilia or muscular dystrophy, good use can be made of a determination of sex early in the pregnancy through amniocentesis of cells from the mother's amniotic fluid.

Another method of prenatal sex determination involves analyzing the blood of preganant women (Grumbach, Conte, and Walknowska, cited in Big step in sex prediction, 1969). The researchers report that successful predictions can be made by the fourteenth week after conception. In this process, the study of at least 1,200 lymphocytes (a class of white blood cells), taken from the pregnant woman, gives a 95 percent chance of finding at least two cells with XY (male) chromosomes. However, this method of using maternal blood samples to determine fetal sex can only prove by indirection that the child is of the female sex—because no XY chromosomes are found. The success of this blood test also demonstrates that fetal cells, as well as oxygen, drugs, diseases, and nutrition, pass through the placental membrane into the mother's blood stream.

A third method of prenatal determination of sex was discussed recently in the *Chinese Medical Journal* (cited in Leff, 1975). This method is somewhat like amniocentesis, but testing can be done much earlier than the sixteenth week of pregnancy. The physician inserts a suction tube into the pregnant woman's cervix and withdraws some of the sloughed-off cells, which can be checked for the sex of the fetus in much the same way as is done in amniocentesis. The Chinese predictions of sex were accurate 93 percent of the time. Researchers in the United States are now trying to copy and improve the Chinese technique. It has been pointed out (Campbell, 1976) that this Chinese technique can have

enormous consequences, for its ultimate purpose is not prediction, but control. In the Chinese researchers' words: "The work was started to help women who desire family planning." These 100 experimental sex predictions resulted in 30 planned abortions. Planned families, fewer people—and evidently "planning" in this case included the sex of the child. But there was one remarkable side-effect of this experiment in rational living. Of the 30 aborted fetuses, 29 were girls. It seems that the availability of sex control led mothers to avoid bearing girls. [p. 86]

The moral and philosophical issues will be discussed later.

Another approach to sex determination requires potential parents to decide *in advance* of conception whether they want a boy or a girl. The scheme exploits the fact that each sperm cell carries either an X chromosome and produces a girl when merged with the X chromosome in the mother's egg, or a Y chromosome and produces a boy if it fertilizes the ovum. In any one male ejaculation there are more Y- than X-bearing sperm. The Y-bearing sperm are sleeker and move faster, but they die sooner than their X counterparts. Also, the Y-bearing sperm are slowed down more than the X-bearing sperm by the normal acidic secretions of the vagina, but they respond more favorably to the alkaline environment of the uterus. Since male babies outnumber female babies by a ratio of 106 to 100, it has been suggested that this uneven ratio results from the faster

165

progress of the lighter Y-bearing sperm through the female reproductive system.

Adapting their technique to these theories, Rorvik and Shettles (1976)[11] recommend proper timing for intercourse in relation to ovulation of the egg, and for taking either an acid (vinegar) or an alkaline (baking soda) douche (depending on which sex is desired). If a girl is desired, intercourse should be preceded by an acid douche, and there should be no further intercourse for two to three days before ovulation. (The reason is that the X sperm can survive for a few days in an acid environment which in the same period will have killed off all the Y sperm.) On the other hand, if a boy is wanted, intercourse should occur as close to the time of ovulation as possible and should be preceded by an alkaline douche, so that the Y sperm will have the best chance of hitting the ovum target.

Rorvik and Shettles report a more than 80 percent chance of success if their instructions are followed carefully. Other researchers are skeptical of Rorvik's and Shettles' reported high rate of success but admit that the method shows theoretical promise. It appears to be generally agreed that their methods will not do any harm—so long as the couple will accept a child of either sex if the method fails.

There now appears to be concern about the increasing use of sex control. Campbell (1976) suggests three general themes to this concern. First, the ultimate effects of sex control on society are profoundly complex and vague. Second, sex control has a definite potential for leading to trouble. Campbell feels that the current tendency is to dwell on the possible positive effects of sex control (such as the elimination of sex-linked genetic defects) without considering the negative effects (such as the obvious biological

[11]Rorvik and Shettles (1976) give specific directions for the techniques of sex determination that are only briefly outlined here.

and social problems that might be created by overstocking the world with boys). Third, sex control, dangerous or not, appears to be inevitable and unstoppable, and this may be the most disturbing theme of all. Campbell concludes his article with some perturbing food for thought: "Some enthusiastic medical engineer is about to let another bawling genie out of the bottle of science. We can congratulate ourselves in advance for having chosen its sex, but that's about it" (p. 91).

Abortion

An abortion occurs when a pregnancy is terminated. If termination occurs spontaneously without outside interference by the mother or physician, it is called either a miscarriage or a spontaneous abortion. It has been popularly believed that miscarriages or spontaneous abortions are nature's way of eliminating abnormal babies, and recent research (Roberts and Lowe, 1975) supports this view. One study of 3,418 fetuses showed malformations to be three times more frequent in fetuses obtained from spontaneous abortions than in fetuses obtained from artificially interrupted pregnancies. Roberts and Lowe conservatively estimate that about three out of four conceptions are lost because of malformations of the developing child. Austin (1972) has this to say about prenatal fetal wastage:

Accumulating evidence suggests that prenatal elimination is in the main an important and valuable provision of Nature. The fact is becoming increasingly clear that a large proportion of resorbed or aborted embryos and fetuses are abnormal, and that their summary disposal is in the best interests of the race. Probably this represents the main way in which disadvantageous features from gene mutation are prevented from being incorporated into the overall hereditary pattern. Indeed if we must grieve over

167

pregnancy losses it should be rather because so many products of anomalous [abnormal] development will succeed in evading this act of natural selection. [p. 134]

There is some evidence that more male fetuses than female fetuses are lost prenatally through spontaneous abortions. It has been estimated (Beatty and Gluecksohn-Waelsch, 1972) that while approximately 130 to 150 males are conceived for every 100 females, only about 106 males are born for every 100 females. The higher prenatal death rate for males is also in agreement with the fact that males, in comparison to females, have a higher death rate during infancy, are less likely to resist infections, and have a shorter life expectancy (Fryer and Ashford, 1972).

It is also possible to terminate a pregnancy through an induced abortion. Since the 1973 Supreme Court decision upheld the right of expectant mothers to have abortions, legally induced abortions have become more common. According to the Supreme Court decision, abortions are permitted, with some restrictions designed to protect maternal health, during the first six months or the first two trimesters of pregnancy. During the last three months or final trimester of pregnancy, abortions are prohibited in some states except when necessary to save the mother's life or health.

Legal approval of abortion, especially in those cases when abortion is performed solely because the mother does not want the child, has opened a Pandora's box of problems and questions that involve social, psychological, and moral considerations as well as further legal issues. One important question, from society's point of view, is whether the fetus has a legal right to be born. If so, at what point in prenatal development does this right begin—at conception, ten days, eight weeks, or six months after conception? If it is accepted that life begins at the moment of conception, does this mean abortion should be regarded, either morally or legally, as murder? Another important question has to do with the right of a woman to control her body and the use of her body, and, also, whether it is psychologically damaging to a woman to undergo an abortion.

Few issues in American history have become the focus of such passionate dispute and personal conflict.[12] A few quotations from a debate on the topic, "Ban all abortions?" (1976), provide the flavor of the arguments on both sides and the intensity of the discussion. In answer to the question, "Why is the Catholic Church seeking a constitutional amendment to prohibit abortion?" Archbishop Joseph L. Bernardin, President, National Conference of Catholic Bishops, replied:

The 1973 Supreme Court abortion decisions have made abortion on demand a fact throughout the United States, with the result that our country now faces a startling and terrifying reality: With the approval of the law, 1 million human lives are destroyed each year by abortion. Considerations of health or economic distress cannot account for all of this. The plain fact is that many of these human lives are destroyed simply because others find it convenient to destroy them.

I think it is important to underscore the fact that the Supreme Court did not legalize abortion in just a few exceptional cases. In effect, it legalized abortion on demand. The 200-year-old tradition of the American people and the Judeo-Christian principles on which this nation was established are clearly opposed to abortion on demand, and a large segment of the American people today are opposed to abortion on demand.

But due to the Supreme Court's decisions, the American people are denied access to the ordinary legislative remedies of such a situation. The only way to correct the error of the Supreme Court decision is to amend the Constitution. [p. 27]

[12]Callahan (1970) provides excellent discussion of the arguments and research evidence both for and against abortion.

Archbishop Bernardin goes on to state that in the legislative process any amendment should be guided by these principles:

First, establish that the unborn child is a person under the law, from conception on. Second, the Constitution should express a commitment to the preservation of life to the maximum degree possible. Third, the protection resulting therefrom should be universal. And fourth, the proposed amendment should give the States the power to enact enabling legislation. [p. 28]

In reply Rabbi Richard S. Sternberger, Chairperson of The Religious Coalition for Abortion Rights, states that his organization opposes a constitutional amendment to outlaw or further restrict abortions for two basic reasons:

We believe very strongly in a woman's right to make her own choice: We're a prochoice organization, not a proabortion organization. We believe that this is a matter of individual conscience—that a woman has to make this choice in consonance with her conscience and with her religious beliefs—and that it is not a legal matter.

Secondly, we believe very strongly in the separation of church and state, and we are very, very concerned about the imposition by law of any theological stance, whatever it be, on the citizens of this country. [p. 27]

In support of this view Rabbi Sternberger goes on to say:

We don't support abortion as a method of family planning. We support education in family planning, but we don't believe that abortion is a technique for family planning.

To repeat: We are not proabortion—we are prochoice. We don't emphasize abortion, but we emphasize the right of choice. We feel that within the first two trimesters where abortions are safe—medically safe, medically feasible—that a woman should have the right to choose concerning her body and the use of her body.

170

I feel that the way to solve many of the problems that we have in this country and in the world is through a program of family planning. People have said this is a racist plot. . . . This is not so. Under the Supreme Court decisions, no one is forced to have an abortion. That is the point—that is why we oppose any legislation that would force anyone to act in contravention of their conscience. [p. 28]

The sharp conflict in these two views makes it clear that the pros and cons of abortion will remain an issue of contention for some time. One thing does appear clear. Knowledge of the stages of prenatal development, such as the fact that after the age of viability at twenty-eight weeks the child is usually capable of life outside the mother's womb, should be an important element of any discussion regarding abortion.

Birth

The discussion of prenatal influences on the unborn child ends with the process of birth, but as has been evident throughout this book the effects of prenatal experiences upon the individual's physical, psychological, and physical development will persist throughout its entire life. To call birth a miracle may sound trite, but there seems to be no other appropriate word to describe the many intricate sequences of events necessary to produce a new human life.

It should be obvious by now that birth is only an event of life rather than the beginning of life. In fact, it is a tradition among many Oriental people such as the Chinese to credit a child with the age of one year on the day of its birth in order to recognize all the growth and development that has already occurred since the time of conception. As one student said when this Chinese tradition was discussed, "It sure does seem like a gyp for us to start a baby again at age zero after all they have already been through before birth." To which an Oriental student responded, "The trouble with Americans is that they never believe anything until they see it!" It is hoped that this will no longer be true of the readers of this book.

Glossary

abortion: termination of a pregnancy spontaneously or through outside interference before the unborn child can survive outside the uterus; spontaneous abortion (also called miscarriage) is termination without outside interference.

afterbirth: the expulsion of the placenta, amniotic sac, and umbilical cord from the mother's body after the birth of the baby.

age of viability: age of seven months or twenty-eight weeks after conception, by which time the fetus is usually capable of independent life and is likely to survive if born.

albino: person with a deficiency of coloring matter resulting in abnormally white skin and hair and pink eyes; results from inheriting two recessive genes for albinism from the parents.

allele: the different forms that a specific gene can take at a particular location on a chromosome.

amniocentesis: the tapping of the amniotic fluid surrounding the unborn child in order to examine skin cells and other substances in the fluid for abnormality.

amniotic sac: membrane filled with amniotic salty fluid that completely surrounds the fetus by eight weeks after conception and acts as a shock absorber. Also known as the "bag of waters."

anoxia: occurs when the amount of available oxygen falls below the requirements of the organism. Sometimes a problem during the birth process.

antibodies: a substance produced in the body in response to an antigen, and possessing the ability to neutralize or react with the antigen.

antigens: a substance capable of forming antibodies when introduced into the bloodstream.

Apgar test: used for assessing the health of a newborn on a scale of zero to two for five categories (appearance [color], heart rate, reflex irritability, activity, muscle tone, and respiratory effort). A score of 10 is perfect, seven is normal, and three or less means the newborn is in a dangerous condition.

blastocyst: fertilized ovum during the second week after conception when it is a hollow ball of cells. Period ends when the blastocyst embeds in the wall of the uterus and becomes an embryo.

bone ossification: the process of converting cartilage to real bone cells that begins about two months after conception.

breech birth: baby presents its buttocks rather than its head at the opening of the birth canal.

cartilage: the tough, elastic, whitish tissue that makes up the initial embryonic skeleton until it is replaced by true bone cells during the process of bone ossification.

catch-up growth: even though a child may be slowed down in growth due to malnutrition or illness, a self-correcting force develops to help the child catch up toward its original growth curve once the missing food is available or the disease ends.

cephalocaudal development: the progression of physical and motor development from head to toe or top to bottom.

chromosome: the beadlike strings of genes present in all cells of the body. Man has 46 chromosomes or 23 pairs, except in the germ cells (sperm or ovum).

congenital defects: abnormalities present at birth resulting from either heredity or the events of prenatal development.

congenital hydrocephalus: excess of fluids collects in the brain cavity when brain cells do not multiply sufficiently, usually as a result of drug, disease, or radiation damage to the brain during the early stages of prenatal development. Also called "water on the brain."

cretin: person characterized by a stunted and malformed body and slow mental development resulting from a prenatal shortage of sufficient iodine to form properly functioning thyroid glands.

critical periods: certain limited periods during the growth and development of an organism when it will interact with the environment in a specific way.

differentiation: developmental trend in which the developing child's body parts become increasingly specific and distinct during the embryonic and fetal periods. Also applicable to the process in which abilities become more distinct and specific after birth.

dizygotic twins: nonidentical fraternal twins resulting from the fertilization of two separate ova released about the same time.

dominant gene: gene for a trait that appears in an individual if paired with a similar gene, and also when paired with a different gene for the trait.

Down's syndrome: a condition characterized by mental retardation and physical abnormalities usually resulting from the presence of three No. 21 chromosomes. Also known as Mongolism.

ectoderm: outer cell layer in the developing embryo from which the skin, sense organs, and nervous system will emerge.

electroencephalogram: a tracing which shows the changes in electric potential produced by the brain.

embryo: term given to the developing child during the six-week period from the end of the second week until the end of the second month after conception. At the end of this period the developing child has taken on the appearance of a human being through the process of differentiation.

endocrine system: made up of the endocrine glands (thyroid, adrenal, and pituitary) that produce internal secretions which are carried by the blood or lymph to the part of the body whose functions they control.

endoderm: inner cell layer in the developing embryo from which the digestive and glandular systems and the lungs will develop.

erythroblastosis fetalis: a disease, which may attack the offspring of Rh-negative women and Rh-positive men, characterized by the destruction of fetal red blood cells by the mother's Rh antibodies.

Fallopian tube: tube attaches at one end to the uterus, and the other end lies free. It functions as the connection between the ovary and the uterus; it is an undulating structure that practically surrounds the ovary in order to pick up the egg as it ruptures from the ovary. Also known as the oviduct.

fertilization: occurs when a sperm released by the male during the act of sexual intercourse merges with the female ovum in one of the Fallopian tubes.

fetology: area of medical science concerned with techniques for diagnosing and treating fetal illnesses and defects.

fetoscope: instrument used to look directly at the unborn child in its mother's uterus to check for defects not apparent in cell analysis; also called endoscope.

fetus: term given to the developing child during the period lasting from the end of the second month after conception until birth.

gene: a unit of a chromosome that gives one particular order in the construction of a human being.

germinal stage: the period of prenatal development lasting from fertilization until the end of the second week after conception.

Glossary

gestation: period of prenatal development.

hereditary defect: a defect that is inherited in the genes or chromosomes from the parents and can be passed on to future children.

heterozygous: condition in which an individual's cells contain different genes for the same trait, and the dominant gene will determine the appearance of the trait.

homozygous: condition in which an individual's cells contain similar genes for a trait so that trait will appear in the individual.

Huntington's chorea: a dominant genetic disease characterized by the onset of nervous-system degeneration in adulthood.

hyperplasia: the stage of brain development during which the number of brain cells increases. Human brain cell division normally occurs during gestation and in the early part of the first year of life.

Liley technique: procedure in which a child affected with Rh disease receives an intrauterine transfusion of blood before birth.

low-birth-weight baby: baby weighing under 5½ pounds or 2,500 grams after a normal period of prenatal development.

meiosis: type of division occurring only in the production of germ cells (ova or sperm) during which each chromosome pair splits and separates so that the resulting ova or sperm contain only 23 single chromosomes.

mesoderm: middle cell layer in the developing embryo from which the musculatory, circulatory, and excretory systems will develop.

methadone: a drug used as a substitute for heroin in the treatment of drug addicts.

methylmalonic acidemia: a genetic disease involving a defect in vitamin B_{12} synthesis resulting in an abnormal build-up of acids in the body, continual vomiting, slow development, and eventual death.

microcephaly: characterized by unnatural smallness of the head and severe mental retardation. Can result from extreme malnutrition or from radiation as well as from a rare recessive gene.

miscarriage: another term for spontaneous abortion; see abortion. The term miscarriage is seldom used medically.

mitosis: process in which a single body cell divides into two exactly equal new parts that contain exactly the same 23 pairs of chromosomes found in the original cell.

Mongolism: see Down's syndrome.

monozygotic twinbirth: very rare occurrence when one twin develops inside the body of its identical twin. Also known as "fetus-in-fetu."

monozygotic twins: identical twins resulting from the same fertilized ovum or egg which later splits into two individuals for some unexplained reason.

morphogenesis: differentiation of the various parts of the body.

multiple birth: the arrival of two or more babies separated by minutes or hours.

myelinization: the process in which a white, fatty substance covers the nerve fibers thus speeding up the transmission of nerve impulses. As the process continues both prenatally and after birth, the child becomes capable of more controlled movement and sensory functions.

neonate: term for a baby during the first month after birth.

ovum: female reproductive cell (also known as the egg), which is the largest cell in the human body.

phenylketonuria (PKU): disease caused by an inherited recessive gene resulting in the inability to metabolize phenylalanine which is a component of many foods.

phocomelia: baby born lacking limbs or with limbs in embryonic stage of development. Often associated with the mother's use of the drug thalidomide during early pregnancy.

placenta: the blood-filled spongy mass that makes it possible for the mother and fetus to exchange materials such as nutrients and waste products. Becomes part of the afterbirth.

postmature infant: baby born two or more weeks beyond the expected arrival date.

potentially pregnant: state of being for any woman of childbearing age who has engaged in sexual intercourse without the use of adequate contraceptive protection (definition taken from "Drugs in pregnancy:are they safe?, 1967).

premature birth: term no longer considered scientifically correct because it does not provide enough information about the characteristics of an individual baby. Term has been replaced by two more descriptive terms: short-gestation-period baby and low-birth-weight baby.

quickening: the first time the mother feels any movement of the fetus within her body.

recessive gene: the subordinate member of a pair of genes whose trait appears only when paired with a similar recessive gene.

retrolental fibrophasia: damage to the cells of the retina in the eye resulting in partial or total blindness sometimes caused by the use of large doses of pure oxygen in an incubator.

Rh factor: "Rh" is an abbreviation for the first two letters of "rhesus" monkey. An inherited factor in human blood causing the blood of Rh-positive people to clump in response to a special serum while the blood of Rh-negative people does not clump.

Rh immune globulin: acts as a vaccine to stop the production of Rh antibodies after an Rh-negative woman gives birth to an Rh-positive child. Commercial name for one gamma globulin is Rhogam.

rubella syndrome: a variety of characteristics such as congenital cataracts, deafness, heart disease, microcephaly, and stunted growth often associated with the mother's infection with German measles or rubella during the early part of her pregnancy.

sex chromatin body: a condensation of nuclear material possessed only by female cells.

sex chromosomes: a single pair (among 23 pairs of chromosomes) that alone determines the individual's sex. Males have an unequal XY pair with the longer of the pair called the X chromosome and the shorter one the Y chromosome. Females possess two similar chromosomes (XX).

sex-linked defect: a kind of genetic defect more frequently occurring in males (XY) since their smaller second Y sex chromosome often does not carry the necessary gene to mask the effect of a recessive gene on the X chromosome.

short-gestation-period baby: baby born early before completing the normal period of thirty-eight weeks of prenatal development.

sickle cell anemia: a hereditary disease caused by a recessive gene that is carried by about 10 percent of American blacks.

singleton: only one baby results from a pregnancy.

spermatozoon: a single male sperm cell necessary for the fertilization of a female ovum.

spontaneous abortion: see abortion.

stillbirth: a baby born dead.

systems-interaction approach: view of human development stressing the continual and progressive interaction between the developing systems of the child and its environment.

Tay-Sachs disease: recessive hereditary enzyme deficiency found almost exclusively among Jews of Eastern European descent. Disease caused by inability of the body to break down fatty materials which accumulate in the nerve cells and result in deafness, blindness, and early death of the child.

teratogen: any agent which produces or raises the incidence of malformations in a population.

teratogenic: factors such as drugs that cause malformations during prenatal development.

teratology: branch of science dealing with malformations. Also called the science of monsters.

testosterone: principal male sex hormone.

thalidomide: a tranquilizer and sedative drug widely prescribed in Europe in the early 1960s that was later found to produce severely deformed children if taken early in pregnancy.

toxemia: the cause is unknown, but the name appears to be a misnomer since there is no evidence that toxemia is actually caused by toxic substances. Depending on the severity of the disorder the symptoms include: high blood pressure, fluid retention, protein in the urine, convulsions, coma.

trisomy: presence of three chromosomes rather than the normal pair usually found on all the 23 locations in a human cell.

umbilical cord: the cord connecting the placenta with the fetus. Baby's lifeline for bringing in food and oxygen and for discharging waste material.

zygote: a fertilized ovum formed by the merging of the female ovum and the male sperm.

References

Adams, J. M., H. D. Heath, D. T. Imagawa, M. H. Jones, and H. H. Spear. Viral infections in the embryo. *American Medical Association Journal of Diseases of Children,* 1956, 92:109–114.

Alter, B. P., S. Friedman, J. Hobbins, M. J. Mahoney, A. S. Sherman, J. F. McSweeney, E. Schwartz, and D. G. Nathan. Prenatal diagnosis of sickle-cell anemia and alpha G-Philadelphia. *New England Journal of Medicine,* 1976, 294:1039–1040.

Ampola, Mary G., Maurice J. Mahoney, Eiichi Nakamura, and Kay Tanaka. Prenatal therapy of a patient with vitamin B_{12}-responsive methylmalonic acidemia. *New England Journal of Medicine,* 1975, 293:313–317.

Antonov, A. N. Children born during the siege of Leningrad in 1942. *Journal of Pediatrics,* 1947, 30:250–259.

Austin, Colin R. Artificial control of reproduction. In Colin R. Austin and Roger V. Short, eds., *Reproduction in mammals,* Vol. 5. Cambridge, England: Cambridge University Press, 1972.

Babson, S. Gorham, Norman B. Henderson, and William M. Clark, Jr. Preschool intelligence of oversized newborns. *Proceedings of the 77th Annual Convention of the American Psychological Association,* 1969, 4:267–268.

Badr, F. M., and Ragaa S. Badr. Induction of dominant lethal mutation in male mice by ethyl alcohol. *Nature,* 1975, 253:134–136.

Ban all abortions? *U.S. News & World Report,* September 27, 1976, pp. 27–28.

Beatty, R. A., and Gluecksohn-Waelsch. Edinburgh Symposium on the Genetics of the Spermatozoan. Edinburgh, Scotland: University of Edinburgh, 1972.

Becker, R. Frederick, and William Donnell. Learning behavior in guinea pigs subjected to asphyxia at birth. *Journal of Comparative and Psychological Psychology,* 1952, 45:153–162.

Bell, Joseph N. When babies go hungry. *Good Housekeeping*, June, 1974, 3:92–93, 168, 170–171.

Benson, R. C., F. Shubeck, W. M. Clark, H. Berendes, W. Weiss, and J. Deutschberger. Fetal compromise during elective cesarean section. *American Journal of Obstetrics and Gynecology*, 1965, 91:645–651.

Berlin, C. M., and C. B. Jacobson. Link between LSD and birth defects reported. *Journal of American Medical Association*, 1970, 212:1447–1448.

Bernard, Harold. *Human development in western culture*. Boston: Allyn & Bacon, 1962.

——. *Child development and learning*. Boston: Allyn & Bacon, 1973.

Berrill, Norman John. *The person in the womb*. New York: Dodd, Mead, 1968.

Big step in sex prediction. *Science News*, 1969, 96:76–77.

Blatz, William Emet. *The five sisters*. New York: Morrow, 1938.

Blinick, George, Robert C. Wallach, and Eulogio Jerez. Pregnancy in narcotics addicts treated by medical withdrawal: the methadone detoxification program. *American Journal of Obstetrics and Gynecology*, 1969, 105:997–1003.

Bowes, Watson A. I. Obstetrical medication and infant outcome: a review of the literature. In Watson A. Bowes, Yvonne Brackbill, Esther Conway, and Alfred Steinschneider, eds., The effects of obstetrical medication on fetus and infant. *Monographs of the Society for Research in Child Development*, 1970, 35 (No. 4):3–23.

Bowes, Watson A., Yvonne Brackbill, Esther Conway, and Alfred Steinschneider. The effects of obstetrical medication on fetus and infant. *Monographs of the Society for Research in Child Development*, 1970, 35 (No. 4):1–49.

Brady, Roscoe O. Hereditary fat-metabolism diseases. *Scientific American*, August, 1973, 229:88–98.

Braine, M. D. S., C. B. Heimer, H. Wortis, and A. M. Freedman. Factors associated with impairment of the early development of prematures. *Monographs of the Society for Research in Child Development*, 1966, 31:1–92.

Brecker, Edward M. *Licit and illicit drugs*. Mount Union, N.Y: Consumers Union, 1972.

Brody, Jane E. Will our baby be normal? *Woman's Day*, August, 1969, pp. 47, 79–81, 99.

——. How doctors can assure more perfect babies. *Woman's Day*, February, 1977, pp. 65, 150, 152, 154.

Bronsted, H. W. Warning and promise of experimental embryology. In Bertrand Russell, ed., *Impact of science on society*, Vol. 6, No. 4. New York: Simon & Schuster, 1955.

Butler, N. R., H. Goldstein, and E. M. Ross. Cigarette smoking in pregnancy: its influence on birth weight and perinatal mortality. *British Medical Journal*, 1972, 2:127–130.

Callahan, Daniel J. *Abortion: law, choice, and morality*. New York: Macmillan, 1970.

Campbell, Colin. What happens when we get the manchild pill? *Psychology Today*, August, 1976, 10:86–88, 90–91.

Carmichael, Leonard. The onset and early development of behavior. In Paul H. Mussen, ed., *Carmichael's manual of child psychology*, Vol. 1. New York: John Wiley, 1970.

Chang, Henry, John C. Hobbins, Gabriel Cividalli, Frederic D. Frigoletto, Maurice J. Mahoney, Yuet Wai Kan, and David G. Nathan. In utero diagnosis of hemoglobinopathies: hemoglobin synthesis in fetal blood cells. *New England Journal of Medicine*, 1974, 290:1067–1068.

Clarke, C. A. The prevention of "rhesus" babies. *Scientific American*, November, 1968, 119:46–52.

Coffey, Victoria P., and W. J. E. Jessop. Maternal influenza and congenital deformities. *The Lancet*, 1959, 2:935–938.

Coleridge, S. T. In Thomas Ashe, ed., *Miscellanies, aesthetic and literary*. London: Bell & Sons, 1885.

Conway, Esther, and Yvonne Brackbill. II. Delivery medication and infant outcomes: an empirical study. In Watson A. Bowles, Yvonne Brackbill, Esther Conway, and Alfred Steinschneider, eds., The effects of obstetrical medication on fetus and infant. *Monographs of the Society for Research in Child Development*, 1970, 35 (No. 4):24–34.

Corner, George Washington. Congenital malformations: the problem and the task. In *Congenital malformations: papers and discussions presented at the First International Conference on Congenital Malformations*. Philadelphia: Lippincott, 1961.

Cravioto, J., E. R. DeLicardie, and H. G. Birch. Nutrition, growth, and neuro-integrative development: an experimental and ecologic study. *Pediatrics*, 1966, 38 (1, Pt. 2, supplement):319–372.

Cruise, M. O. A longitudinal study of the growth of low birth weight infants. I. Velocity and distance growth, birth to 3 years. *Pediatrics*, 1973, 51:620–628.

Davison, A. N., and J. Dobbing. Myeliniation as a vulnerable period in brain development. *British Medical Journal*, 1966, 22:40–45.

Dayton, Delbert H. Early malnutrition and human development. *Children*, 1969, 16:210–217.

Denenberg, V. H. Stimulation in infancy, emotional reactivity, and exploratory behavior. In David C. Glass, ed., *Neurophysiology and emotion*. New York: Rockefeller University Press and Russell Sage Foundation, 1967.

Developmental psychology today. New York: CRM/Random House, 1975.

Drillien, C. M., and R. W. B. Ellis. *The growth and development of the prematurely born infant.* Baltimore: Williams and Wilkins, 1964.

Drugs in pregnancy: are they safe? *Consumer Reports,* August, 1967, 32:435.

Eastman, N. J. Editorial comment. *Obstetrical and Gynecological Survey,* 1959, 14:34–36.

Ebbs, J. H., F. F. Tisdall, and W. A. Scott. The influence of prenatal diet on the mother and child. *Milbank Memorial Fund Quarterly Bulletin,* 1942, 20:35–36.

Etzioni, Amitai. Doctors know more than they're telling you about genetic defects. *Psychology Today,* November, 1973, 7:26–29, 31, 35, 36, 137.

Fitzgerald, H. E., and J. P. McKinney. *Developmental psychology: studies in human development.* Homewood, Ill: Dorsey Press, 1970.

Forbes, H. S., and H. B. Forbes. Fetal sense reaction: hearing. *Journal of Comparative Psychology,* 1927, 7:353–355.

Four viruses vindicated from causing birth defects. *Science News,* 1974, 105:20.

France, Anatole. *A little Pierre* (J. L. May, trans.). New York: Dodd, Mead, 1925.

Frazier, T. M., G. H. Davis, H. Goldstein, and I. Goldberg. Cigarette smoking: a prospective study. *American Journal of Obstetrics and Gynecology,* 1961, 81:988–996.

Friedmann, Theodore. Prenatal diagnosis of genetic disease. *Scientific American,* November, 1971, 225:34–42.

Fryer, J. G., and J. R. Ashford. Trends in perinatal and neonatal mortality in England and Wales, 1960–1969. *British Journal of Preventive and Social Medicine,* 1972, 26:1–9.

Graham, M. Intrauterine crying. *British Medical Journal,* 1919, 1:675.

Gregg, N. M. Congenital cataract following German measles in the mother. *Transactions of Opthamologist Association of Australia,* 1941, 3:35–46.

Greulich, W. W. Growth of children of the same race under different environmental conditions. *Science,* 1958, 127:515.

Haggard, H. W., and E. M. Jellinek. *Alcohol explored.* Garden City, N.Y.: Doubleday, Doran, 1942.

Hanson, James W. Unpublished paper, 1977.

Hanson, James W., Kenneth L. Jones, and David W. Smith. Fetal alcohol syndrome: experience with 41 patients. *Journal of the American Medical Association,* 1976, 235:1458–1460.

Hardy, Janet B., and E. David Mellits. Does maternal smoking during pregnancy have a long-term effect on the child? *The Lancet,* 1972, 4:1332–1336.

References

Harrell, R. F., E. Woodyard, and A. E. Gates. *The effects of maternal diet on the intelligence of offspring: a study of the influence of vitamin supplementation of the diet of pregnant and lactating women on the intelligence of their children.* New York: Bureau of Publications, Teachers College, Columbia University, 1955.

Hegel, Georg F. W. *Philosophy of mind* (W. Wallace, trans.). Oxford: Clarendon Press, 1894.

Henahan, John. Mom's couple of drinks per day may produce an abnormal child. *Medical Tribune,* 1977, 18:1, 9.

Hobbins, John C., and Maurice J. Mahoney. In utero diagnosis of hemoglobinopathies: technic for obtaining fetal blood. *New England Journal of Medicine,* 1974, 290:1065–1067.

Holden, R. H., E. B. Man, and W. P. Jones. Maternal hypothroxinemia and developmental consequences during the first year of life. Paper presented at the Meeting of the Society for Research in Child Development, Santa Monica, California, March, 1969.

How mother's smoking affects her child. *Science News,* 1973, 104:168.

Huffman, J. W. Pregnancy. *Encyclopedia Britannica,* 1974, 14:968–984.

Human conception in test tube. *Science News,* 1973, 104:168.

Hurley, L. S. The consequences of fetal impoverishment. *Nutrition Today,* 1968, 3:2–10.

Hutchings, D. E., and J. Gibbon. Effects of vitamin A excess administered in late pregnancy on discrimination learning in offspring. *Proceedings of the 79th Annual Convention of the American Psychological Association,* 1971, 6:211–212.

Jalavisto, E. Parental age effects on man. In G. E. W. Wilstenhomle and M. O'Connor, eds., *The lifespan of animals.* Boston: Little, Brown, 1959.

James, William *The principles of psychology,* Vol. 1. New York: Holt, 1890.

Janerich, Dwight T., Joyce M. Piper, and Donna M. Glebatis. Oral contraceptives and congenital limb-reduction defects. *New England Journal of Medicine,* 1974, 291:697–700.

Joffe, J. M. *Prenatal determinants of behavior.* London: Pergamon Press, 1969.

Johansson, B., E. Wedenberg, and B. Westin. Measurement of tone response by the human fetus. *Acta Otolaryng,* 1964, 57:188–192.

Jones, Kenneth L., and David W. Smith. Recognition of the fetal alcohol syndrome in early infancy. *The Lancet,* 1973, 2:999–1001.

Jones, Kenneth L., David W. Smith, Ann P. Streissguth, and Ntinos Myrianthopoulos. Outcome in offspring of chronic alcoholic women. *The Lancet,* 1974, 1:1076–1078.

Kan, Yuet Wai, Mitchell S. Golbus, and Richard Trecartin. Prenatal diagnosis of sickle-cell anemia. *New England Journal of Medicine,* 1976, 294:1039–1040.

Kato, T. Chromosome studies in pregnant rhesus macaque given LSD-25. *Diseases of the Nervous System,* 1970, 31:245–250.

Keating, Thomas R. Rare birth at Riley Hospital. *Indianapolis Star,* January 19, 1973, p. 25.

Knobloch, Hilda, and Benjamin Pasamanick. Prospective studies on the epidemiology of reproductive casualty: methods, findings, and some implications. *Merrill-Palmer Quarterly,* 1966, 12:27–43.

Kolodny, Robert C., William H. Masters, Robert M. Kolodner, and Gelson Toro. Depression of plasma testosterone levels after chronic intensive marijuana use. *New England Journal of Medicine,* 1974, 290:872–874.

Kraemer, Duane C., Gary T. Moore, and Martin A. Kramen. Baboon infant produced by embryo transfer. *Science,* 1976, 192:1246–1247.

Laurence, K. M. Fetal malformations and abnormalities. *The Lancet,* 1974, 6:939–942.

Leff, D. N. Boy or girl: now choice, not chance, amniocentesis raises new ethical questions for doctors. *Medical World News,* December 1, 1975, 16:45–46.

Liley, A. W. Intrauterine transfusion of halmolytic disease. *British Medical Journal,* 1963, 2:1106–1110.

Liley, Helen Margaret Irwin. *Modern motherhood.* New York: Random House, 1967.

Lilienfeld, A. M., B. Pasamanick, and M. Rogers. Relationship between pregnancy experience and the development of certain neuropsychiatric disorders in childhood. *American Journal of Public Health,* 1963, 45:637–643.

Lipsitt, L. P., and N. Levy. Pain threshold in the human neonate, *Child Development,* 1959, 30:547–554.

Locke, John. *Essay concerning human understanding* (1690). Philadelphia: Kay & Troutman, 1849.

Lovell, Kenneth. *Introduction to human development.* Glenview, Ill.: Scott, Foresman, 1971.

Lubs, H. A., and F. H. Ruddle. Chromosomal abnormalities in the human population: estimation of rates based on New Haven newborn study. *Science,* 1970, 169:495–498.

Marijuana-hashish epidemic and its impact on United States security. Hearings before the Subcommittee to Investigate the Administration of the Internal Security Act and Other Internal Security Laws of the Committee on the Judiciary, United States Senate, 93rd Congress, Second Ses-

References

sion, May 9, 16, 17, 20, 21, and June 13, 1974. Washington, D.C.: U.S. Government Printing Office.

Matthews, H. B., and M. G. derBrucke. Normal expectancy in the extremely obese pregnant woman. *Journal of American Medical Association,* 1938, 110:554–559.

McClearn, Gerald E. Genetic influences on behavior and development. In Paul H. Mussen, ed., *Carmichael's manual of child psychology,* Vol. 1. New York: John Wiley, 1970.

McGlothlin, W. H., R. S. Sparkes, and D. O. Arnold. Effect of LSD on human pregnancy. *Journal of American Medical Association,* 1970, 212:1483–1487.

McLaren, A., and D. Michie. Studies on the transfer of fertilized mouse eggs to uterine foster-mothers. I. Factors affecting the implantation and survival of native and transferred eggs. *Journal of Experimental Biology,* 1956, 33:394–416.

Mendelson, Jack H., John Kuehnle, James Ellingboe, and Thomas F. Babor. Plasma testosterone levels before, during and after chronic marijuana smoking. *New England Journal of Medicine,* 1974, 291:1051–1055.

Methadone addiction in babies. *Science News,* 1972, 101:170.

Montagu, M. F. Ashley. *Prenatal influences.* Springfield, Ill.: Charles C Thomas, 1962.

——. *Life before birth.* New York: New American Library, 1964.

Morrison, F. J. Maternal impressions. *Virginia Medical Monthly,* 1920, 47:127.

Murphy, D. P. The outcome of 625 pregnancies in women subjected to pelvic roentgen irradiation. *American Journal of Obstetrics and Gynecology,* 1929, 18:179–187.

Mussen, Paul H., John J. Conger, and Jerome Kagan. *Child development and personality.* New York: Harper & Row, 1974.

Nash, John. *Developmental psychology: a psychobiological approach.* Englewood Cliffs, N.J.: Prentice-Hall, 1970.

Neel, J. V. The effect of exposure to the atomic bombs on pregnancy termination in Hiroshima and Nagasaki: preliminary report. *Science,* 1953, 118:537–541.

Nora, J., and A. Nora. Editorial. *New England Journal of Medicine,* 1974, 291:649–650.

Pasamanick, Benjamin, and A. M. Lilienfeld. Association of maternal and fetal factors with development of mental deficiency. 1. Abnormalities in the prenatal and paranatal periods. *Journal of the American Medical Association,* 1955, 159:155–160.

Peckham, C. H., and R. W. King. A study of intercurrent conditions observed during pregnancy. *American Journal of Obstetrics and Gynecology*, 1963, 83:609–624.

Performance in school linked to birth weight. *Quarterly Newsletter of the National Institute of Education*, 1974, 1:1.

Pregnant women warned against pain relievers. *New York Times*, October 25, 1976, p. 16L.

Prenatal sex hormone levels: a possible link to intelligence. *Science News*, 1972, 101:8.

Proceedings, Third National Conference on Methadone Treatment, U.S. Public Health Service Publication No. 2172. Washington D.C.: U.S. Government Printing Office, 1971.

Rhodes, A. J. Virus infections and congenital malformations. *Congenital malformations: papers and discussions presented at the First International Conference on Congenital Malformations*. Philadelphia: Lippincott, 1961.

Roberts, C. J., and C. R. Lowe. Where have all the conceptions gone? *The Lancet*, 1975, 6:498–499.

Robinson, R. J., and J. P. M. Tizard. The central nervous system in the new born. *British Medical Journal*, 1966, 22:49–55.

Rogers, Dorothy. *Child psychology.* Belmont, Calif.: Brooks/Cole, 1969.

Rorvik, David M., and Landrum B. Shettles. *Choose your baby's sex.* New York: Dodd, Mead, 1976.

Rugh, Roberts, and Landrum B. Shettles. *From conception to birth: the drama of life's beginnings.* New York: Harper & Row, 1971.

Salk, Lee. Thoughts on the concept of imprinting and its place in early human development. *Canadian Psychiatric Association Journal*, 1961, 11:295–305.

——. Mother's heartbeat as an imprinting stimulus. *Transactions of the New York Academy of Science*, 1962, 24:753–763.

——. The role of the heartbeat in the relation between mother and infant *Scientific American*, May, 1973, 228:25–29.

Sameroff, A. J. Early influences on development: fact or fancy? *Merrill-Palmer Quarterly*, 1975, 21:267–294.

Schulman, C. A. Sleep patterns in newborn infants as a function of suspected neurological impairment of maternal heroin addiction. Paper presented to the Meeting of the Society for Research in Child Development, Santa Monica, Calif. 1969.

Shank, Robert E. A chink in our armor. *Nutrition Today*, 1970, 5:2–11.

Shapiro, Sam, Edward R. Schlesinger, Robert E. L. Nesbitt. *Infant, perinatal, maternal and childhood mortality in the United States.* Cambridge, Mass.: Harvard University Press, 1968.

Sheridan, M. D. Final report of a prospective study of children whose

References

mothers had rubella in early pregnancy. *British Medical Journal,* 1964, 2:536–539.

Sickle cell anemia detected in fetuses. *Science News,* 1976, 109:325.

Siegel, Morris. Congenital malformations following chickenpox, measles, mumps, and hepatitis. *Journal of the American Medical Association,* 1973, 226:1521–1524.

Siegel, M., and H. T. Fuerst. Low birth weight and maternal virus diseases: a prospective study of rubella, measles, mumps, chickenpox, and hepatitis. *Journal of American Medical Association,* 1966, 197:680–684.

Simpson, W. J. Preliminary report on cigarette smoking and the incidence of prematurity. *American Journal of Obstetrics and Gynecology,* 1957, 23:808–815.

Smart, Mollie S., and Russell C. Smart. *Children: development and relationships.* New York: Macmillan, 1972.

Smith, D. J., and J. M. Joffee. Increased neonatal mortality in offspring of male rats treated with methadone or morphine before mating. *Nature,* 1975, 253:202–203.

Smoking, carbon monoxide, and the fetus. *Science News,* 1972, 102:424.

Solkoff, N., S. Yaffe, D. Weintraub, and B. Blase. Effects of handling on the subsequent development of premature infants. *Developmental Psychology,* 1969, 1:765–768.

Sontag, L. W. The significance of fetal environmental differences. *American Journal of Obstetrics and Gynecology,* 1941, 42:996–1003.

——. War and the fetal-maternal relationship. *Marriage and Family Living,* 1944, 6:3–4, 16.

——. Implications of fetal behavior and environment for adult personalities. *Annals of the New York Academy of Sciences,* 1966, 134:782–786.

Sontag, L. W., and H. Newbery. Normal variations of fetal heart rate during pregnancy. *American Journal of Obstetrics and Gynecology,* 1940, 40:449–452.

Sontag, L. W., and R. F. Wallace. The effect of cigarette smoking during pregnancy upon the fetal heart rate. *American Journal of Obstetrics and Gynecology,* 1935, 29:77–83.

Spelt, David K. The conditioning of the human fetus in utero. *Journal of Experimental Psychology,* 1948, 38:338–346.

Stechler, Gerald. Newborn attention as affected by medication during labor. *Science,* 1964, 144:315–317.

Stevenson, H. C. Learning in children. In P. H. Mussen, ed., *Carmichael's manual of child psychology,* Vol. 1. New York: John Wiley, 1970.

Stone, Lawrence J., and Joseph Church. *Childhood and adolescence: a psychology of the growing person.* New York: Random House, 1973.

Strean, L. P., and A. Peer. Stress as an etiologic factor in the development of cleft palate. *Plastic and Reconstructive Surgery*, 1956, 18:1–8.

Subak-Sharpe, Genell J. Is your sex life going up in smoke? *Today's Health*, August, 1974, pp. 50–53, 70.

Surgeon General, U.S. Public Health Service. *Smoking and Pregnancy*. U.S. Government Printing Office, 1971.

Swine flu: did Uncle Sam buy a pig in a poke? *Consumer Reports*, 1976, 41:495–498.

Tanner, J. M. Physical growth. In Paul H. Mussen, ed., *Carmichael's manual of child psychology*, Vol. 1. New York: John Wiley, 1970.

Taussig, H. B. The thalidomide syndrome. *Scientific American*, 1962, 107:29–35.

Test-tube babies: now a reality? *Science News*, 1974, 106:37.

Thompson, W. R., and J. A. Grusec. Studies of early experiences. In P. H. Mussen, ed., *Carmichael's manual of child psychology*, Vol. 1. New York: John Wiley, 1970.

Thong, Y. H., R. W. Steele, M. M. Vincent, S. A. Hensen, and J. A. Bellanti. Impaired in vitro cell-mediated immunity of rubella virus during pregnancy. *New England Journal of Medicine*, 1973, 289:604–606.

Unnecessary illness, The. *Time*, September 24, 1973, p. 86.

Vore, David A. Prenatal nutrition and postnatal intellectual development. *Merrill-Palmer Quarterly*, 1973, 19:253–260.

Waddington, Conrad Hal. *Principles of development and differentiation*. New York: Macmillan, 1966.

Weathersbee, Paul S. Heavy coffee intake, miscarriages linked. *Muncie Evening Press*, October 16, 1975, p. 19.

Whitehead, J. Convulsions in utero. *British Medical Journal,* 1867, pp. 59–61.

Winick, Myron. *Malnutrition and brain development*. New York: Oxford University Press, 1976.

Winick, M., and P. Rosso. Head circumference and cellular growth of the brain in normal and marasmic children. *Journal of Pediatrics*, 1969, 74:774–778.

Witkin, Herman A., A. Mednick Sarnoff, Fini Schulsinger, Eskild Bakkestrom, Karl O. Christiansen, Donald R. Goodenough, Kurt Hirschhorn, Claes Lundsteen, David R. Owen, John Philip, Donald Rubin, and Martha Stocking. Criminality in XYY and XXY men. *Science*, 1976, 193:547–555.

World Health Organization. *Public health aspects of low birth weight*. Third Report of the Expert Committee on Maternal and Child Health. World Health Organization: Technical Report Series, 1961, No. 217.

Wyden, B. Growth: 45 crucial months. *Life*, December 17, 1971, pp. 93–95.

References

Yerushalmy, J. Infants with low birth weight born before their mothers started to smoke cigarettes. *American Journal of Obstetrics and Gynecology,* 1972, 112:277–284.

Zimmerman, David R. Your family's health. *Ladies' Home Journal,* October, 1976, 93:78.

Index

Index

external growth failure, 137
internal growth failure, 137
prognosis, 137-138
relation to smoking, 94-98
LSD (lysergic acid diethylamide), 118-122

Malnutrition, 67-72
Marijuana, 117-118
  male fertility, effect on, 118
Maternal characteristics:
  age, 85-86
  emotional state, 80-85
  fatigue, 92
  size, 86-87
  See also Alcohol, Blood oxygen level, Coffee, Radiation, Rh factor incompatibility, Smoking
Maternal-fetal connection, 22-23, 26, 102-104
  drugs and diseases, effect on, 102-104
  emotions, effect on, 81-82
  indirect connection, 17-18
  superstitious beliefs about, 15-18
  transfer of immunity, 23, 103
Measles, 125-127
Meiosis, 144, 150
Mesoderm, 27
Methadone, 18, 116-117
Methylmalonic acidemia, 62-63
Microcephaly, 93
Miscarriage. See Spontaneous abortion
Mitosis, 144
Mongolism. See Down's syndrome
Multiple births, 43-46
  fraternal or dizygotic twins, 44
  frequency of, 43
  identical or monozygotic twins, 43
  monozygotic twinbirth, 45-46
  problems of, 44-45
Mumps, 125-127
Myelinization, 51, 57, 77-78

Neonate, 49
Nutrition, prenatal, 63-67
  diet, importance, 63-64

effect on time of conception, 64-66
fallacies, 72-75
influence on brain development, 77-79
optimal pregnancy weight gain, 79

Oversized babies, 140
Ovum, 19

Phenylketonuria (PKU), 143, 145-147
Phocomelia. See Thalidomide
Placenta, 21-23
Polyhydramnios, 50-51
Postmaturity, 140
Pregnancy, length of, 42-43
Pregnant woman, potentially, 109-110
  advice on drug usage, 121-122
"Prematurity," 43, 133, 139-140
  causes, 133-134
  different treatment of prematures, 138-139
  See also Low-birth-weight infant, Short-gestation-period infant
Prenatal treatment of disorder, 62-63

Quickening, 31

Radiation, prenatal, 92-94
Recessive genes, 145-146
Retrolental fibrophasia, 135
Rh factor incompatibility, 87-90, 160
  erythroblastosis fetalis, 87-88
  frequency of occurrence, 87
  Liley technique, 89
  Rh immune globulin, 89
Right to be born normal, 133
Rubella. See German measles

Self-righting tendency, 61-63
Sensory development, 47
  hearing, 52-57
  smell, 51-52
  taste, 50-51
  touch, 48-50
  vision, 57-58
Sex chromosomes, 31, 42, 148-150

193

Index

The Child before Birth

Designed by R. E. Rosenbaum.
Composed by Vail-Ballou Press, Inc.,
in 11 point VIP Palatino, 3 points leaded,
with display lines in Palatino bold.
Printed offset by Vail-Ballou Press on
P & S offset, 60 pound basis.
Bound by Vail-Ballou Press.
Color plates and jacket printed by
Simpson/Milligan Printing Co., Inc.

Library of Congress Cataloging in Publication Data
(For library cataloging purposes only)

Annis, Linda Ferrill, 1943–
  The child before birth.

  (Cornell paperbacks)
  Bibliography: p.
  Includes index.
  SUMMARY: Examines prenatal development and factors influencing the unborn
child, such as nutrition, maternal characteristics and experiences, drugs, and
diseases.
    1. Fetus.   2. Prenatal influences.   3. Fetus—Diseases. [1. Fetus.   2. Prenatal
influences]
  I. Title.
RG600.A55   618.3'2   77-3112
ISBN 0-8014-1039-8
ISBN 0-8014-9168-1 pbk.